the
Birth
Book

the Birth Book

PERSONAL STORIES, FACTS AND ADVICE

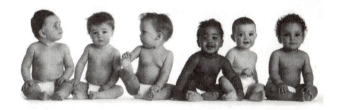

CAROL BARBAR

with JANE PALMER

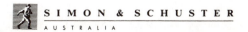

SIMON & SCHUSTER
AUSTRALIA

The information in this book is not intended to be a substitute for medical care and advice. You are advised to consult a health-care professional with all matters relating to your health, including matters that may require diagnosis or medical attention.

All the stories in this book are true-life accounts, although some people have chosen to remain anonymous. To protect these individuals' privacy, some names and places have been changed and minor alterations made to their stories.

THE BIRTH BOOK
First published in Australia by Carol Barbar in 1998
This revised and updated edition published in 2001 by
Simon & Schuster (Australia) Pty Limited
20 Barcoo Street, East Roseville NSW 2069

A Viacom Company
Sydney New York London Toronto Singapore

National Library of Australia Cataloguing-in-Publication data:

Barbar, Carol.
The birth book: personal stories, facts and advice.
Includes index.
ISBN 0 7318 0934 3
1. Childbirth – Anecdotes. 2. Labour (obstetrics). I. Title.

618.4

Cover design by Gayna Murphy, Greendot Design
Internal design and typesetting by DiAgn
Set in Adobe Garamond 11.5 pt on 15 pt
Printed in Australia by Griffin Press

10 9 8 7 6 5 4 3 2 1

Foreword

Carol Barbar in *The Birth Book* has done what no obstetrics textbook can ever do – she has given childbirth the humanity and depth of emotion it deserves. By allowing ordinary women to tell their stories of birthing, we begin to see clearly how every delivery is a unique experience – no two women will have the same feelings or the same experience, and even the same woman will experience each birth differently. This book will help women to understand that there is no 'set' way to have a baby, and that indeed there are many options available. Reading the stories of these ordinary women will make the 'mum-to-be' aware that she can question and she can actively contribute to how the delivery of her child will occur. By sharing these women's experiences, Carol allows the reader to broaden her visions and understanding of birth. Above all, this book will share with you the tears and the elation, the pain and the wonder of the miracle of birth, and you may find yourself wishing for (or remembering) that moment when all pain is forgotten, and you hold your child in your arms and you are indeed a mother.

Sue McCully MB, BS
Mother of two

Contents

part one Pregnancy   1

Acknowledgments

This book is dedicated to:

Sylvia from the Early Childhood Centre, Marrickville, for giving me the push I needed to begin writing; my sister Patricia, for her support and encouragement; Mary Barber, for her useful criticism, as well as her encouragement in not giving up when the going got tough; and Cheryl Morrone, who first started me writing about my experiences.

I also wish to thank the following for their involvement in the production of this book:

Cindy Lord, editor of *Sunshine Baby* magazine; Dr Sue McCully, Marrickville Medical Centre; Carolyn Parfitt, former editor of *Mother and Baby* magazine; Lynn Keen, Breastfeeding Columnist, 'Welcome Home Australia', the Institute of Children's Literature (USA), and midwife Annie Popelier of the Australian Society of Independent Midwives.

Introduction

Giving birth to my first child was a dismal experience that robbed me of that exquisite joy of having a newly delivered baby. I was too drugged to enjoy my newborn and too inexperienced to realise my lack of knowledge had contributed to such painful contractions.

I have written this book to let other first-time mums avoid what I went through and help all mums have a better labour. (How I wish this book had been available when I was a novice at childbirth!)

Now the mother of nine children, I am delighted to be able to say that it is knowledge (which I share with you in this book) that has enabled me eight more 'enjoyable' labours, so different from my first, bad experience, which I now know could have been avoided.

One thing I wish to convey is that pregnant women are beautiful. The inner and outer beauty of the promise of life helps us get through the nausea, aches and pains. A feeling of fulfilment is gained that cannot be had from any other source.

I wish to thank all the women and professional people who let me interview them for this book. Without them, there would not be one.

Not all the beliefs, practices and approaches to pregnancy and birth expressed in the stories are necessarily those I hold myself. However, in the interests of helping as many women as possible understand the birth experience and to know their choices, they have been included in the book.

I also apologise to those people whose stories I did not use. Their material was good, but my manuscript grew too large – perhaps big enough for a second volume!

Our ninth baby, Lily, is now almost eleven months old and, despite all the work, is a precious and beautiful little darling, who brings us great joy and love.

part **one**

Pregnancy

Welcome to one of the most exciting events in your life. Pregnancy and birth is a time of great change, and you will be experiencing an amazing mixture of emotions. Giving birth can be painful, elating, frightening and joyful all at once. Although this book is primarily about childbirth, it is hard to remove the pregnancy stage when discussing birth, especially when some things in pregnancy directly effect the way in which you may ultimately give birth. This section is not intended as a comprehensive guide to pregnancy, and for many important details on pregnancy it will be necessary to speak to your health-care professional. A list of books on pregnancy is also supplied at the back of this book.

As you read through the text, certain words are in bold type. This means they can be found in the glossary at the back of the book.

As early as five to seven days after conception, the tiny embryo embeds itself firmly into your uterine wall, where it will be nourished and continue to grow for the next nine months. Pregnancy hormones are released into your bloodstream. These account for those early pregnancy symptoms, such as a strange metallic taste in your mouth, tender breasts and a need to urinate more frequently. Almost straight away you may feel extreme tiredness and even nausea. The tiredness is your body's way of forcing you to take it easy in those early days when it is so important to be stress-free. The earlier you find out that you are pregnant, the earlier you can care for yourself and your baby, by avoiding substances such as alcohol and nicotine, and reducing stressful situations that may harm the developing baby. Stress and caffeine are now known to increase the chances of early miscarriage, while a nutritious diet, appropriate exercise and relaxation are highly beneficial for both mother and baby.

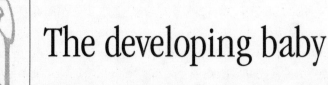

The developing baby

Pregnancy may seem a long time when you are waiting for your baby, but when you consider the amazing process that is going on, it seems hardly any time at all. Once the ovum has been fertilised by the sperm, growth begins. The fertilised cell divides rapidly over the next few days and by around the seventh day is implanted in the **uterus**, which then provides nutrients for the embryo. As the embryo is firmly establishing itself in the lining of the uterus (endometrium), the **placenta** begins to grow. The cells of the embryo begin to group, and within four to six weeks the embryo has a circulatory system, a nervous system, a developing brain and liver, and is developing arms and legs. By the ninth week the baby is called a fetus.

Throughout this time the fetus is supplied with blood, oxygen and nutrients from the mother's blood supply, although her blood never directly comes in contact with the fetus. The fetus is genetically different from the mother and would be rejected by the mother's body if blood was supplied directly to it. Everything is filtered through the placenta and transferred via the umbilical cord to the baby. This continues until the baby is born.

By eight weeks most of the baby's organs and structures are formed, and by four months the baby is moving and stretching, although all work is still done for the baby through the placenta. At approximately 40 weeks the baby begins its descent into the birth canal to be born. At birth, the baby's heart takes over from the placenta, and blood flows to the baby's lungs to allow it to breathe.

Placenta

The placenta is an amazing organ that permits the exchange of nutrients between the mother and baby and helps with the removal of waste products. The blood supplies of mother and baby pass very closely in the placenta, but do not mix. The placenta supplies oxygen to the baby. It also acts rather like a sieve, allowing very small things to pass across to the baby, such as viruses or some medications, while other things are prevented from reaching the baby. The placenta is also responsible for producing a range of hormones that help maintain the pregnancy. During pregnancy, the placenta is usually attached high up on the wall of the uterus. Once the baby is born, the uterus shrinks and the placenta peels off the wall of the uterus and is born. A healthy placenta is reddish brown in colour, looks like a piece of raw liver and is about the size of a dinner plate.

Jesenka's pregnancy diary

Weight chart

Onset of pregnancy	67.0 kg
16 weeks (4 months)	71.5 kg
20 weeks (5 months)	71.0 kg
21 weeks	72.5 kg
23 weeks (5^1/$_2$ months)	73.5 kg
29 weeks (6^1/$_2$ months)	74.5 kg
30^1/$_2$ weeks	75.0 kg
32^1/$_2$ weeks (7^1/$_2$ months)	75.5 kg
36 weeks + 2 days (8 months + 2 days)	75.0 kg
37 weeks + 2 days	76.5 kg
39^1/$_2$ weeks	75.5 kg
40 weeks (9 months + 1 day)	77.0 kg

Towards the end of November

I think I might be pregnant! I feel different, and have feelings in my stomach I don't normally have.

But since I've had several false alarms, I'm not counting on it because I always end up disappointed when I get my period. But this time the feeling in my stomach is different, and my stomach looks bloated.

I am also feeling a bit nauseated, so with all these symptoms I am pretty certain I'm pregnant, but Phillip (my husband) and I have decided to wait before visiting a doctor, just to make sure.

2 weeks later

I go to my doctor and have my urine tested. The result comes out 'sort of positive' — one very dark line, but the other going across is very faint, turning what would have been a negative into an almost positive. The doctor says she can't say for certain that I'm pregnant, but neither can she say that I'm not. So she suggests one more blood test, just in case.

The day has come for my test results. I phone the doctor to discover I am indeed pregnant! I get off the phone and excitedly tell Phillip, who is equally delighted. After six and a half months of trying, I am now exactly six weeks pregnant.

For the next three months, I suffer a lot of tiredness and nausea, and I crave creamed corn mixed with ice cream. Also pickles and dips.

2 months pregnant

I am now needing to wear maternity dresses. I don't feel comfortable in regular clothes any more. (My stomach seems to be growing very quickly, making it uncomfortable for me to wear anything even slightly tight.)

At my doctor's visit, we discussed options for the birth. I decided to go with the birth centre, as I wanted to avoid the hospital where I gave birth seven years ago. I don't want this birth to take place in that operating theatre (which is how I view the labour ward), so my doctor has written me a referral.

I phoned the birth centre today and they asked me to attend an information night before I book with them.

I have attended that information night and have definitely made up my mind to have the baby at the birth centre, but now have to book in quickly before all their available places are taken.

My first visit is arranged.

16 weeks pregnant

I have decided to have my daughter with me for the birth, and am told I can do this as long as she has her own support person. I have some forms to fill in, and my blood pressure is checked (it is 125/80). My stomach is felt and I get to hear the baby's heartbeat. After this I go to another part of the hospital to have some blood tests done.

20 weeks

I have decided to decline an **ultrasound** offered to me at eighteen weeks as I feel there is nothing wrong with the baby, and also because the **midwife** told me the long-term effects of ultrasounds are unknown.

I hope that the new knowledge I have acquired during this pregnancy is going to make this birth less painful than when I had Merita. Back then I didn't know about giving birth. As soon as I went into the labour ward I lay on the bed, causing myself a lot of pain, and more work for my body. I am hoping to give birth without pain-relieving drugs, as I don't want this baby to feel the side effects.

Previously at each visit I was told I would be seen by a midwife, so am surprised that today I am being seen by a man. But the results are good and my blood pressure is 125/65.

24 weeks

This is my third check-up. I am curious as to why I wasn't seen by a midwife at the previous visit, so I ask about it. The midwife tells me that the man who saw me is the **obstetrician**, who examines the women to make sure they are fit to give birth in the birth centre. I feel relieved that I am fit, and that my previous pregnancy wasn't too complicated.

My blood pressure is 120/70 and my **fundal height** is 27. This is surprising, because I am still only 24 weeks. (My fundal height should only be 24.) I now feel I might be carrying twins, so ring my mum to ask if there are any twins in our family. 'Yes,' Mum replies. 'Two of your aunts are twins.' (I had, in fact, been told this ten years earlier, but it didn't seem important at the time, so slipped my mind. Now it does seem important, as I seem to be getting so big so quickly.) I ask the midwife if she can discover more than one baby. She searches with the heart monitor, then feels my stomach, but tells me that although she is not certain, she thinks there is only one baby.

27 weeks + 2 days

I have now been going to pregnancy and childbirth classes and have been told about **Braxton Hicks contractions**. They are like tightenings of your stomach, happening from about twenty weeks on, we are told. I realise I have indeed been feeling these tightenings, but thought it was my stomach stretching. One evening I actually felt a pain so strong that I thought I was about to give birth. It's much too soon, I worriedly thought, until realising it was just one of those Braxton Hicks pains. Straight afterwards, my baby gave me several strong kicks.

27¹/₂ weeks

As the days progress, I am becoming more and more convinced I am having twins.

Tonight I feel as though two babies are turning at the same time.

I was woken several times last night because of arms and legs hitting and kicking me from all directions.

I am now exactly 28 weeks pregnant (if I carry to term I have only 12 weeks to go)

I am six and a half months pregnant, but feel about seven or eight months. I am so big and heavy I tend to waddle when I walk. I am also experiencing heartburn, and sitting on the floor is becoming painful. I am also experiencing pains, which might be **contractions**, and am having trouble sleeping at night, but apart from this I feel well.

28 weeks + 2 days

At this, my fourth check-up, I am given a glucose test: I have to drink a lime-flavoured drink then wait an hour before having some blood taken. After this, the midwife checks my blood pressure and takes a vaginal swab. She mentions that I look a bit thrushy and tells me the test will also show if I have other bugs present. The midwife feels my stomach, but tells me she can only feel two poles (that is, head and bottom). She tells me to forget the idea I might be having twins. I haven't gained any weight since my last check-up and still weigh 73.5 kilograms.

28¹/₂ weeks

Today I phoned the birth centre to get the results from my antenatal tests. All of them are okay except my iron levels, which are a bit low. They have dropped from 11.7 at the beginning of my pregnancy to 10.6 at the moment.

29 weeks

It is now one week since my last check-up and my weight has gone up to 74.5 kilograms (I have gained 1 kilogram in one week).

29+ weeks

I was woken several times last night with pains in my lower stomach, each time needing to go to the toilet, but could only pass a small amount of urine. Today I am still getting the pains, which are even more frequent.

1 pm: I am now timing the pains, as I feel they are coming too often. In fact, they're coming every five minutes and are starting to worry me. I phone the birth centre and they say it sounds like premature labour and to come straight in.

At the labour ward, I first need to give a urine sample, then have a monitor attached. My blood pressure is also taken. Half an hour later, the monitor is taken off and the doctor presses on my stomach, which is quite painful. He takes a vaginal swab and examines my **cervix** to see if I have begun to **dilate**. Fortunately I haven't and he tells me it doesn't look like labour, although it could be a urinary tract infection. The doctor tells me if a urinary infection isn't treated quickly it can bring about premature labour, so prescribes some antibiotics, telling me to come back on Monday morning for the results.

30 weeks

My fifth visit. My blood pressure is 120/70 and my fundal height is 30. At my last check-up, my baby was in the **breech** position [bottom facing down], but is now head down with its feet towards my ribs.

30+ weeks

Today I visit my local doctor to make sure my urinary infection has completely cleared. I am now finding I need lots of rest as, if I walk or even stand for extended periods, I begin to feel pains.

31 weeks + 1 day

I go to my doctor because of the pain I am feeling while walking. She examines me and tells me I have an inflammation at the front of my pelvis that is causing this pain. She tells me I have a condition known as diastasis symphysis pubis [see next page for information] and a support belt will probably ease the pain. She tells me I need to see a physiotherapist to have the belt fitted.

Diastasis Symphysis Pubis (also known as Pubis Symphysitis)

Your symphysis pubis is the joint in the middle of your pelvic girdle. By placing your fingers low on your pubic bones and pressing down firmly, you should be able to feel what appears to be solid bone. But, in fact, what you are feeling are two sides of your pelvis fused together to create a joint which is almost immovable. During pregnancy, these joints undergo a gradual change, due to the influence of pregnancy hormones, and become a little more elastic, therefore allowing the symphysis pubis to open up somewhat during childbirth, giving the baby more room from which to emerge. Normally this process should cause the pregnant woman no pain at all; however, in the condition known as *diastasis symphysis pubis* or *pubis symphysitis*, the woman does experience pain, and sometimes even extreme pain.

31 weeks + 2 days

Today, after my pregnancy preparation classes, I visit the physiotherapist. She fits me with an elastic support belt, which gives me immediate relief from my pain.

32 1/2 weeks

I am now finding that if I wear the belt until bedtime it allows me to walk without feeling much pain. But I am still unable to rush or run about.

33 weeks

Today at 8 am I was in the bathroom when I felt something trickling between my legs. I cleaned myself up, then spent most of the day rushing around buying things I need for the baby.

Since lunchtime today I have been having regular, painless contractions every 20 to 30 minutes and have been feeling shaky and unable to eat. This is how I felt while in labour with Merita, so am thinking I might be in labour. (I was trying to hold it off until I had bought all the things I needed.)

I phone the birth centre and am told it sounds like labour, but because I still have seven weeks to go am told the baby is too premature to be delivered at the birth centre. I have to go to the labour ward. I now rush around quickly getting things together in my hospital bag, then Dad drives Phillip and me to the hospital. After an examination I am told I am not dilating, but should have an ultrasound tomorrow to see how much fluid is around the baby. I am asked to stay overnight to make sure I am not contracting, but Phillip and I feel that since nothing is happening and the baby is all right, we might as well go home. A different doctor now comes, who tells me I can go.

37 weeks

I had a dream last night that I gave birth in the birth centre. My dream was very clear and I saw myself having twins. The first baby was a big boy, followed shortly by a girl.

38 1/2 weeks

I am having very strong contractions and seem to be in labour. Some of my contractions are seven to ten minutes apart and my cervix is now 1.5 centimetres dilated. But after a while nothing seems to be happening.

39 weeks

Once again I am experiencing contractions, this time three to five minutes apart, but, when I go to the birthing centre, nothing happens. The contractions stop and I don't dilate any further.

Almost 40 weeks

I have had a **show** and over the past few days have had quite a few pains. Last night I had very painful contractions several times during the night, but none of them were regular.

Today at my check-up everything was fine. It's the sixth, and the midwife said that if I haven't given birth by the sixteenth I should have an ultrasound to make sure the baby is all right. Then if I haven't had the baby within five days after the ultrasound, I will be induced with a prostaglandin gel. I do believe I will have given birth by then – hopefully within the week – so I won't need an **induction**.

4O weeks + 8 days

I am now eight days overdue. Today I went for an ultrasound at 2 pm.

I asked the nurse what sex the baby is, but she couldn't tell because its legs were folded underneath it. The baby's heartbeat and my contractions were also monitored. Everything was fine, so we went to pick up Merita from school.

Jesenka went into labour naturally. Her story continues in Part 2.

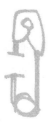

Nausea and vomiting during pregnancy

Unfortunately, one of the drawbacks in early pregnancy can be nausea. Hard as it is to eat when you feel sick, this is often the only way to relieve the nausea. You will need to eat small amounts frequently, as often as five or six times a day.

Nausea is usually at its worst first thing in the morning and in the early evening, when your blood sugar levels are low or you are feeling tired. Bland foods such as banana, creamed corn or a hot milk drink may temporarily ease your nausea if your stomach is particularly queasy. To stabilise your blood sugar try to eat starchy foods, such as crackers, bread and pasta, whenever you can manage it. Dry toast or crackers with a cup of tea may help to counter queasiness in the morning and late at night. Acupressure bands (also known as 'seasickness' bands), which are worn on your wrist, have been known to help. Also, ginger tablets or ginger tea and vitamin B6 may help to settle your stomach.

If the smell of food cooking is a big problem, and it often is, it will be an enormous help if you can get someone to do your cooking during those couple of months while your nausea is at its worst. Not eating will definitely make you feel worse, so be prepared to eat something.

Nausea usually begins around week six of your pregnancy, when pregnancy hormones begin to rise steeply. By week fifteen, most women are over their nausea.

For some women, nausea and vomiting are so severe that nothing seems to stop their constant sickness. In these extreme cases, a trip to the doctor may become necessary so that you can be given an injection and/or tablets – ones which are safe to take while pregnant – to ease your nausea.

I took an anti-nausea medication from the time I was six and a half weeks pregnant with my fourth child, as I had previously been vomiting up to twenty times per day, consequently ending up on a **drip** after becoming dehydrated. The medication, although not removing my nausea, had eased it a little and reduced the amount of vomiting down to a third. This type of medication can be what breaks that vicious cycle of vomiting and sickness, or, if not, can reduce the extent of your vomiting.

Please remember that it is of course better to avoid all medication while pregnant, especially during the first few weeks of your pregnancy, during which time your baby's limbs and organs are developing. Also, anti-nausea drugs do not work for everyone.

If nausea is a persistent problem for you and is causing you to become depressed, here is a simple course of action that may temporarily take your mind off it. Recall something you normally do which totally absorbs your mind – something from which you gain great satisfaction. For example, if you love reading, writing, drawing or a craft, do so. Become totally absorbed in what you are doing and distract your mind from the sickness you feel. This can make you forget, at least for a while, those dreadful pregnancy symptoms. It can diminish and even remove your perception of your nausea. Of course, it will probably return once you stop your enjoyable activity, but hopefully by then this distraction will have changed your frame of mind.

Wendy's all-day morning sickness

I suffered morning sickness for the first sixteen weeks of my pregnancy – and it wasn't just morning sickness, it went on all day.

I spent most of my time lying on the couch feeling cranky and depressed. People would tell me to sleep away the afternoon, but if I did this I would wake up feeling even more depressed.

I had found out I was pregnant very early in the pregnancy and was initially very excited. But by week eight I went into a real crisis, not being sure about the whole thing.

At nine weeks I was lying in bed talking to my husband, Richard, about my fears and about how I wasn't sure if being pregnant was the right thing for me – when suddenly I felt a little twinge of something, a little spark I am certain was the baby. Consequently, I lost any doubts I had and now felt relieved and pleased at my decision to go ahead.

Finally over my nausea, the next five months were wonderful. I engaged my own midwife, who had been recommended as someone who really encouraged women to be strong and fit during their pregnancy. I was still swimming a kilometre at the pool two weeks before my baby was born, and climbing the mountain behind our home. But, by the time I was nearly nine months pregnant, I had become too heavy and had to stop.

Wendy's baby was in face presentation. Her story continues in Part 5.

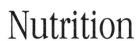

Nutrition

Eating well can help you feel better during pregnancy, give you a glowing skin, increase your energy levels and give you a better outlook on life. Well-nourished women have fewer problems during pregnancy, a decreased chance of birth defects, a reduced incidence of premature birth and respond better to the stress of labour. Well-nourished women's bodies are stronger and their tissues more elastic. Ensuring a well-balanced diet with plenty of protein, iron, calcium, zinc, folic acid, fibre and water is one of the best things a pregnant woman can do for herself and her baby.

A baby's development relies upon its mother's nutritional intake. Many people think that babies get all the nutrients they need from their mothers, even if their mothers eat poorly. This is an unfortunate misconception. While babies are able to use some of the nutrients stored in their mother's bodies, they cannot gain enough of the nutrients they need this way.

Women often ask if they should take vitamin and mineral supplements during pregnancy. Generally, it is better to gain the necessary nutrients from food rather than pills. The exception is folic acid. It is recommended that all women planning pregnancy should take a folic acid supplement, as it is believed to help prevent spina bifida in the baby. The recommended intake is 500 micrograms daily one month prior to falling pregnant and for the first three months of the pregnancy. Some women will choose to take a multivitamin/mineral supplement during pregnancy. It is important to ensure that this type of supplement has been designed for pregnancy. Some supplements contain high doses of certain vitamins which can be harmful to the baby.

Pregnant women should eat freshly prepared food. Foods that have been stored for longer than twelve hours have an increased risk of carrying the Listeria bacteria. If a pregnant woman develops a Listeria infection, it can be transmitted to the baby and can cause miscarriage, premature birth, stillbirth or severe illness in a baby after birth. Other strategies to help avoid a Listeria infection include avoiding raw or undercooked meats, seafood and eggs. Cooking kills the Listeria bacteria, so hot food should be freshly cooked and served piping hot. Also avoid soft cheeses such as camembert, brie and ricotta.

Exercise in pregnancy

During pregnancy, active women often wish to continue with their exercise routine. For others, pregnancy signals a time to improve their lifestyle. For these women, beginning exercise during pregnancy is desirable, as moderate physical activity has major health benefits. Regular exercise is preferable to intermittent activity. In the past, concerns were raised as to the safety of exercising during pregnancy, and it was common for various restrictions to be placed on women with regard to exercise. However, as the research evidence grows, these restrictions are lifting and a more personalised approach is being adopted. The emerging picture is that in most cases there is no need for healthy women to change their exercise program during **conception** and early pregnancy, although some adaptations are required as the pregnancy advances. Prior to commencing any exercise program, it is wise to seek the advice of a midwife or doctor. It is also of benefit to see a qualified fitness professional, as they can offer guidelines and a training program to suit the individual woman and her pregnancy.

The benefits of exercising during pregnancy include: increased body awareness, increased endurance, improved posture, less fatigue, improved muscle tone, improved body image and shortening of the active phase of labour. Exercise can also aid in the prevention of **gestational diabetes**, lessen the physical discomforts associated with pregnancy and increase a woman's sense of wellbeing, Physically fit women are less likely to have **forceps** and **caesarean** births and will recover more quickly after birth.

When exercising during pregnancy, it is important to follow some simple guidelines:

- If bleeding, cramping, faintness, dizziness or severe joint pain occurs, stop exercising and consult a midwife or doctor.
- Avoid lying flat on your back after sixteen weeks of pregnancy.
- Exercise sensibly at a comfortable intensity and do not exercise to exhaustion or at an anaerobic (breathless) pace.
- Avoid overheating. This is particularly important in the first trimester when the baby is most vulnerable to high temperatures. Wear light, comfortable clothing, drink plenty of water, avoid exercising in hot weather or overheated rooms, and do not exercise during illness or fever.
- Avoid any sport where there is a risk of an abdominal blow, e.g. downhill skiing, horse riding, contact sports.
- Avoid holding your breath during exercise.
- All exercise should be accompanied by an appropriate warm-up and cool-down session.

Exercise during pregnancy is not recommended if a woman has:

- pregnancy-induced hypertension
- **ruptured membranes**

- ◎ an **incompetent cervix**
- ◎ vaginal bleeding
- ◎ interuterine growth retardation
- ◎ a multiple pregnancy.

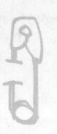

Weight gain

Ahealthy weight gain during pregnancy ranges between 8 to 18 kilograms. The amount a woman gains is dependent on her weight prior to the pregnancy. If a woman is underweight, she needs to gain more weight than a woman in the normal weight range. If a woman is overweight, ideally she will gain less than the average. Gaining weight is a normal, essential part of being pregnant. When a woman's weight gain is within the recommended range, the incidence of low birth-weight babies is reduced. Low or inadequate weight gain during the second half of pregnancy is associated with an increased risk of premature birth.

It is important to focus on healthy eating, not on how many kilograms have been gained. Pregnancy is not a time to try to lose weight, but neither is it necessary to 'eat for two'. What is needed is a well-balanced diet. Just remember, weight gain during pregnancy is individual: some women gain more and some gain less, and this is what is right for them.

Carol's eighth pregnancy

Right from the start it had been a difficult pregnancy. The first four to sixteen weeks involved constant nausea, extreme tiredness and vomiting several times most days. I also felt unsupported, but a great calmness filled my entire pregnancy and everything about me slowed right down.

Since I hadn't gained weight until I was five and a half months pregnant, I was expecting my smallest baby yet. For the whole nine months my appetite was almost nonexistent, so altogether I gained only 7.5 kilograms, but I needed to eat frequently to keep the nausea at bay.

By the end of my pregnancy I was having such trouble breathing I could no longer sleep through the night. My craving to meet and hold my baby had become so strong I became extremely depressed two weeks before my due date. Nothing interested me any more except my baby. I wasn't enjoying my seven other children, I no longer liked reading (except about babies) and I no longer enjoyed my hobby of writing.

On Mother's Day, one week before my due date, it became even worse. I thought I could not stand being pregnant for even one day longer. Surprisingly, it seemed the waiting ended up being for my own good. When I eventually went into labour, things had been done that otherwise wouldn't have been. The freezer was stocked with pre-prepared food, rooms had been scrubbed that never normally got scrubbed, and things needing immediate attention were attended to. (Things not easily done with a newborn.)

Carol had a slow start to her labour but a quick birth. Her story continues in Part 3.

Donna's first pregnancy

I worked as a computer operator for a large company until four weeks before our baby's due date, thinking that I'd have a whole month to get ready for the baby. But things didn't go as I'd expected. I had gained 18 kilograms and I was beginning to feel very uncomfortable due to swelling in my ankles. The girls at work had been great, bringing buckets of cold water for my feet, but unfortunately it didn't help – I still couldn't get into my shoes.

Then, at 36 weeks, not long after my last day at work, I had a sudden burst of energy and began running up and down the stairs of our home to prepare for our baby. Not satisfied with this, I was also spring-cleaning our entire house, leaving nothing undone.

At 38 weeks, my obstetrician said to me; 'Your swelling is getting worse. You must go home and rest or I'll put you into hospital.' Apart from the swelling, everything was fine and the baby was in the right position for delivery.

Donna went into labour that evening. Her story continues in Part 2.

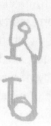

Swelling and fluid retention during pregnancy

Around 50 to 80 per cent of women develop swelling during pregnancy. This swelling, in the absence of a rise in blood pressure, is considered normal. It is known as physiological oedema of pregnancy and usually only involves the lower limbs, although it can occur in the fingers and in the face. Pregnant women often notice that the rings on their fingers become tight. Swelling during pregnancy develops slowly. Interestingly, women who have swelling in pregnancy without rising blood pressure tend to give birth to larger babies than those women who have no swelling in pregnancy. Most women who develop **pre-eclampsia** (see page 20) develop swelling, but not always. Swelling associated with pre-eclampsia can appear suddenly. However, it is very difficult to tell the difference between physiological oedema of pregnancy and the swelling associated with pre-eclampsia. Swelling by itself is common and does not mean that the pregnant woman is at risk of developing blood-pressure problems.

Julia's story

Seven weeks into my pregnancy, I began to feel a little off-colour. Within a week, this queasy feeling had turned into 24-hour nausea, my only relief being when I actually vomited. Feeling dreadful continued until I was five months pregnant. I was extremely relieved when it finally stopped. But then, seven weeks later, something else happened.

I started noticing my hands were swelling and had to take all my rings off. At about the same time, I also came down with something known as **carpal tunnel syndrome**, whereby I felt pins and needles in my fingers all the time. I was told by the birth centre to watch for any sign of sudden swelling. Fortunately, after this my pregnancy continued fairly uneventfully – until one week before my baby was due.

It was a Friday morning and I was at work as usual. A friend commented, 'Your face looks fat today.' Remembering what the birth centre had said about sudden swelling, I rang them and was told to come in. When I arrived it was discovered that my blood pressure had gone up to 126/96. This concerned the midwife, who got me to lie on a bed for half an hour. I soon began to worry that I would be admitted into the labour ward for an induced birth.

Half an hour later, my blood pressure was still high, so we went to the labour ward where a monitor was strapped across my stomach to check the baby's condition. I was on the monitor for an hour. The baby didn't seem to be affected and my blood pressure had now dropped to 110/80, so I was allowed to go home. But, before I went, I was ordered not to do anything – which meant I couldn't go back to work. As well as this, I now had to have my blood pressure monitored every two days at the birth centre.

Julia went into labour two days later. Her story continues in Part 2.

Donna's second pregnancy

My pregnancy with this baby was totally different from my first. For the first three months I suffered morning sickness and felt just terrible. Eating and drinking didn't ease my constant nausea.

A month after I had recovered from the nausea, I began swelling, mainly in my hands, feet and legs. By the time I was six months pregnant it was really bad. Also at around six months I began to get varicose veins and was prescribed support pantyhose, which helped quite a lot. Apart from the swelling, my pregnancy wasn't too bad – that is, until two weeks before my due date. Now my blood pressure went up and I had to be admitted to hospital.

I was kept in for half the day so my blood pressure could be checked every hour or so. The staff told me to relax when I got home, because I hadn't been getting enough rest during the day.

Donna had a fast birth the next day. Her story continues in Part 2.

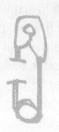

Pre-eclampsia

As mentioned above, during later pregnancy, especially the last ten weeks, swelling as a result of fluid retention can be common. This is not serious unless it is accompanied by high blood pressure and protein in the urine. If you have these symptoms, you may be developing pre-eclampsia (toxaemia). Treatment for pre-eclampsia is usually bed rest and sometimes medication to control blood pressure. This is done to prevent the development of **eclampsia**, a life-threatening condition for both mother and baby, usually necessitating emergency delivery of the child.

Dianne's first pregnancy

Because of an **incompetent cervix**, I had a **cervical suture** inserted when I was sixteen weeks pregnant. Pregnant at 32, this was my first baby and I was unprepared for the possibility of anything other than a natural vaginal delivery. Unfortunately, this wasn't to be the case!

My cervical stitch was removed with great difficulty after 36 weeks, as it had become entangled. Then, at 37 weeks, I developed high blood pressure of 150/90. This, coupled with the fact that I had very large amounts of protein in my urine and swelling of my hands and feet, meant that I was suffering from pre-eclampsia. The doctor decided to admit me straight away.

Following doctor's orders, I went straight home, collected my bag, then took myself back to the hospital by taxi. I was put to bed and given drugs to reduce my still-rising blood pressure. My husband, Brett, joined me later. I continued to rest in bed for the rest of the day and most of the next, but by the following afternoon it was discovered that my blood pressure was not stabilising.

'You are going to have to be induced tomorrow morning,' the doctor told me, 'and if that doesn't work you'll be having a caesarean.'

Dianne was induced the next day. Her story continues in Part 4.

More than one

Discovering you are having two babies can be a shock or a pleasant surprise; three and possibly four can be equally delightful, if a little overwhelming. Twins run in families, so you may already have been aware of the possibility of a multiple birth. Sometimes relatives do not think to pass on that there are twins in the family, and it may not be obvious, because twins do not always appear in every generation. Multiple births are on the increase, partly due to fertility drugs and in vitro fertilisation programs, but also because more women are older when they are having their babies (the chances of giving birth to identical twins increases after the age of thirty-five).

Multiple births are often discovered at the first ultrasound. Pregnancy with twins or more may not be that different from single-baby pregnancies, although your pregnancy will be regarded as high risk and multiple babies often do not go full term. Most mothers carrying more than one baby will be cared for by an obstetrician. The obstetrician will want you to have frequent check-ups and monitoring to ensure your health and that all the babies are growing well and remaining healthy.

Many women comment on feeling greater nausea and fatigue when carrying more than one baby. Also, they tend to feel and look very pregnant much earlier than single-birth pregnancies. Taking extra care with health and nutrition, and resting when you feel you need it, will help with nausea and fatigue and also help you carry the babies longer. Many twins are born around 36–37 weeks. Some come earlier. In the event that your obstetrician thinks your babies may come very early, you may be given injections of steroids, such as betamethasone, to help mature the babies' lungs as early as possible.

Twins are either identical or non-identical. Identical twins grow from the same egg and share a placenta, although they have separate **amniotic sacs**. They are always the same sex. Non-identical (fraternal) twins grow from two different eggs, have different sacs and a placenta each. They can be a boy and girl or the same sex.

Jen's surprise

With my first pregnancy I was really healthy, thoroughly enjoying the experience, and at the end had a perfect little boy weighing 3600 grams. With my second pregnancy, which ended in a miscarriage at fourteen weeks, I suffered morning sickness from three weeks onwards, so when, in my third pregnancy, the severe nausea began at around four weeks, I immediately thought the worst. I suffered chronic nausea 24 hours a day and at around ten weeks ended up in hospital with dehydration. Because of my fears, I arranged to have an ultrasound at twelve weeks, which was ultimately a roller-coaster ride of emotions.

I arrived for the ultrasound having not drunk enough liquid, so when the technician tried to perform the ultrasound she was unable to find any sign of a fetus and asked if I had had the pregnancy confirmed by the doctor. I was devastated. She then suggested I go and drink as much water as possible and come back in half an hour. My husband and I were convinced at this stage that I had once again miscarried, so when we returned for the ultrasound and the technician began to giggle, we thought something very odd was going on. That is when the bomb was dropped, and all I can say now is, it's a good thing I was lying down at the time. Not only was everything fine and I was pregnant, but I was having twins! I laughed and cried excitedly.

The morning sickness disappeared at eighteen weeks and from then on my pregnancy went fairly smoothly. I had the usual heartburn and would occasionally get a racing heart and shortness of breath, feeling faint and nauseous. I was told this was due to my small frame and the twins' limbs pressing on my chest cavity due to space restrictions. It was frightening the first few times, but I soon discovered that if I changed positions and relaxed it would not last for long.

Jen's twins arrived at 37¹/₂ weeks. Her story continues in Part 5.

Jasmine's bonus

My third pregnancy had been difficult right from the start. Having suffered morning sickness from an earlier stage than is usual for me, the nausea was also stronger than with my previous pregnancies. As well as this, from two months I was getting crampy pains, and my stomach was a lot bigger than I thought it should be. At fifteen weeks, a routine blood test at the hospital came back abnormally high. This indicated a possible problem with our baby. I was worried sick and began imagining the worst possible scenario. I cried a lot over the next few days and continued to worry until an ultrasound three weeks later.

Now eighteen weeks pregnant, imagine my shock, relief and disbelief to discover not one healthy baby, but two! Both were doing well, and were the right size for dates. No wonder my stomach was growing so fast! I kept myself very busy for the rest of my pregnancy, looking after my husband, two children and our house and garden. My doctor gave me check-ups every two weeks once it was known I was pregnant with twins. An induction was to be done once I reached 38 weeks, if I got that far, and I was very much hoping to reach full term.

Jasmine was induced at 37¹/₂ weeks. Her story continues in Part 5.

Kuini's third pregnancy

This is the story of my twins, Hamish and James. We were living in New Zealand and had Julia, who was three years old, and Helen, eighteen months, when we decided to come over to Australia for a working holiday.

We were planning to buy a van and travel all over Australia for two years, then return to New Zealand in time for Julia's schooling. So we sold our home and stored the furniture. The house was no longer ours. And then I had this feeling I was pregnant. My partner, Pat, didn't believe me. I went to the doctor. I was indeed pregnant but I was extremely tired, which was different from my pregnancies with Helen and Julia.

The day before we were to fly to Australia I was six weeks pregnant and didn't want to go on the holiday any more. I felt a need to stay back in New Zealand with my family, but Pat still wanted to go, so we flew over anyway. From the moment we arrived in Sydney, Pat's personality changed.

At the time we were staying with my brother, who lives in the eastern suburbs of Sydney, and I was still breastfeeding our youngest daughter Helen. The first thing I did when we arrived in Australia was book myself a midwife. By the time I was three months pregnant I went to my midwife for my first antenatal check-up. Everything was fine. It hadn't yet been confirmed I was pregnant with twins, but all along I had had this feeling I was, so during my first visit I said to her, 'Look, I think I'm having twins.'

The midwife's reply to me was, 'Oh no, your womb is so much bigger because you've had other children.' But I still had this strong feeling I was carrying two babies. In the meantime, Pat and I were very unsettled. We shifted house seven times.

To cut a long story short, when I was about five months pregnant, I walked out on Pat with our daughters Helen and Julia. We went to a woman's refuge, and there I phoned my family in New Zealand to organise a flight back home. But the airlines wouldn't accept me because I looked so big. I was still only five months pregnant but I looked about nine months and they wouldn't even try to book me. 'Well, okay,' I thought, 'I'll just have to stay here then.'

The refuge was horrible. We only stayed there five weeks, but it felt more like a year. I was grateful to have a place to stay, but it was highly stressful and traumatic, and I had always been used to a comfortable standard of living.

The refuge was for women with children who had suffered domestic violence, so all these women had come from terrible circumstances. The only light-hearted times were when the refuge workers went home each night and we were left alone. We would sit and talk about our abuse stories, which was very therapeutic for us. It was really nice to be able to talk things over and share things with people who understood.

After five weeks, the Department of Housing gave my children and me a place to live. A few of my friends from the refuge came with me to look at it, but even while we were there a criminal was breaking into one of the back rooms. So we were allocated another house. When I first went to look at it I really felt comfortable, believing I could be happy to give birth there.

Now that we were settled into our new home, I started having antenatal check-ups again, as I hadn't had any while I had been staying in the refuge. I also started going to a doctor, because I could no longer afford the home birth. I thought I would be going through the hospital system, giving birth at a birth centre. By now I was more than 30 weeks pregnant and looked like a whale. While I was walking down the street, people would stop and stare. Even I couldn't get used to how big I was. But it still wasn't confirmed I was pregnant with twins.

The first time I saw the doctor I said to him, 'Look, I think I'm pregnant with twins,' but the doctor didn't believe me. He wanted me to have an ultrasound, which I wouldn't do, as I don't believe in them. I asked the doctor if he would use a horn to find the two different heartbeats. But instead he replied, 'We no longer do this.'

Over the next few weeks, every time I saw this doctor the babies would kick like crazy in front of him. It was very obvious I was pregnant with twins. I really looked it. By my third visit, when I was 34 weeks, the doctor said he wanted to induce me at 38 weeks. When I asked him why, he said, 'Well, it's the procedure with twins.' It was at this point I knew I didn't trust him.

I had cancelled the midwife when I thought I was going back to New Zealand, so now I contacted her again and we made arrangements so I could pay off the fee on time payment. She was very understanding about it.

The same day I walked out of the hospital I went to the birth centre next door and asked one of the nurses if she could use the horn to find the two heartbeats. The nurse did use it, and she did find the two heartbeats.

Finally having my belief confirmed was incredible. I was 34 weeks pregnant and felt absolute joy. The happiness I felt hearing those words, 'You're having twins,' was like a light bursting inside me. Then I also burst into tears because I was a single mum, struggling and on my own, and about to give birth to two more children. But then on the way home I really felt God had blessed us with these babies when we already had two, so I decided to phone Patrick, who was in New Zealand having a holiday with his parents. We agreed to try once more. Patrick was thrilled when I told him I was pregnant with twins.

Pat arrived three weeks before the birth, and that's when I started feeling that the second baby would be born dead. Whenever friends or visitors came over I would always be talking about the second baby being stillborn. I was also frequently praying that I would accept it. I didn't understand why I was feeling this way, but really believed it would happen.

Everyone thought I was morbid. Patrick believed me, though, so we discussed whether we should go to the hospital, whether we should tell the midwife, or what we should do. After lots of discussion we decided to just leave it be – that it was meant to happen, and to just accept it. We didn't even tell the midwife.

Kuini gave birth at home. Her story continues in Part 5.

Not the usual thing

Pregnancy can bring about some unexpected events, and unexpected events can happen during pregnancy. These stories show that, with proper care, you can have a normal birth despite appendicitis, dog bites and pneumonia.

Susan's nausea

The first three months of my pregnancy were great. I wasn't feeling sick and I hadn't slowed down in any way. I didn't feel fat, and friends were continually telling me how wonderful I looked.

Then, one Friday night when I was twelve weeks pregnant, I started to feel nauseated. I had felt so well up until then that I began to suspect it wasn't related to the pregnancy. By the next morning I was still feeling ill, but went in to work anyway, as I was the only one with the keys and had to open the shop. Once someone else arrived, I left work and went straight to the doctor. I suggested to him that it may be appendicitis, but the doctor told me I was constipated and to go home and relax. I wasn't happy with his diagnosis.

By 12 pm that day I was feeling so dreadful that I had my husband, John, take me straight to the hospital. Nobody seemed to be taking me seriously. They knew I was in pain and that something could be wrong, but I was left to wait for six hours before I was seen by a doctor. Finally a surgeon examined me, and immediately said I had to be rushed upstairs for an emergency appendectomy.

The rest of my pregnancy was fine and I had no more complications, so I did go back to work for three days a week. At 38 weeks I was feeling wonderful. Pregnancy was not preventing me from going about as usual.

Susan went into labour naturally. Her story continues in Part 4.

Jane's pregnancy after miscarriage

I had wanted another child for ages. After Joshua's birth, I chose to study and establish my career in midwifery. By the time we decided that we should try for another child, Joshua was nine years old. I was so excited and expected that I would fall pregnant easily. You can imagine the disappointment when month after month my periods occurred. Ten months later, the line on the pregnancy test window appeared. I did not believe it at first. I had to do the test three times before I would allow the positive result to sink in. I was bursting to tell everyone immediately, but being a whole four weeks pregnant, I tried to refrain. This lasted until I was six weeks pregnant – when I could wait no longer.

I approached my chosen midwives (and good friends) to check on their availability. Their excitement mirrored my own. However, I had this feeling that I was not really pregnant. It was odd, as I had all the symptoms, but this feeling persisted. By the time I was twelve weeks pregnant, I chided myself for being silly and started to relax. Two days later, when I went to the toilet there was a honey-coloured discharge on the toilet paper. This sinking, devastating feeling descended. I tried to rationalise what I saw, but I knew something was wrong. I went to bed trying to dismiss it, but I didn't sleep a wink. The next day I went to work in a daze. I saw one of my midwives and explained what had happened. She offered to try to find the baby's heartbeat with a doppler (a small, hand-held ultrasound). She tried and tried but to no avail. I justified this by telling myself that she couldn't find the heartbeat because it was too early in the pregnancy. I took her advice and went home and rested.

The discharge continued. I knew in my heart that the pregnancy was not to be. On the fifth day I decided to have an ultrasound – I had to know for sure what was happening. I bumped into a fabulous obstetrician as I was waiting for the ultrasound. She said that if there was any problem I was to get the ultrasonographer to call her. I can still remember the heightened anxiety I felt as I waited my turn for the ultrasound. The ultrasonographer took 30 seconds to do the ultrasound and she looked at me and confirmed my worse fears. She explained that there was only a gestational sac and no baby present (known as a blighted ovum). I was numb. The obstetrician took me aside and told me and Frank, my partner, our options. I could have a curette or wait for the pregnancy to end naturally. I chose the latter. The obstetrician gave me her contact numbers and instructed me to call if I needed to. I informed my midwives – I felt supported and safe.

I was now thirteen and a half weeks pregnant. I went to bed that night and said to myself, 'Okay, it is time to end this.' I woke in the wee hours to find the bed soaked with blood and fluid. I was experiencing abdominal cramping. I got up several times through the night and passed large blood clots in the toilet. I sent Frank to work – I needed to be alone. The bleeding continued and became heavier. I started to estimate the blood loss, as it seemed excessive. I was in floods of tears. One of my midwives telephoned to see how I was and we discussed what was happening. On her advice I contacted the obstetrician. The obstetrician confirmed that my blood loss seemed excessive and that a curette was advisable. She organised my admission to hospital, the theatre time and a private room where I knew the midwives. I couldn't have asked for better care. I went to the hospital around lunchtime and was home in the early evening.

The next day I felt empty. I have never cried so much in my life. Bright and cheery flowers arrived from my midwives. I looked at them every day and drew some support. The midwives called to see how I was. It was tough going, but I got through it. The hardest part was when I returned to work and had to care for pregnant women and women with their babies.

We had a follow-up appointment with the obstetrician. She debriefed us on our experience, on what she had found and the impact on future pregnancies. She explained that we could try for another baby as soon as we felt we wanted to. As it had taken a while to fall pregnant, I wanted to try again as soon as possible. I took vitamins and herbal preparations and tried to prepare myself emotionally for another pregnancy.

We waited one menstrual cycle before trying again. One month later, around the time when my period was due, we were having a dinner party. I thought that I might do a pregnancy test, as I wanted to drink some wine if I was not pregnant. You can imagine my surprise when the test proved positive. I was in total denial. I waited another 24 hours and then repeated the test, which was, of course, positive. I then told Frank – I don't think he believed me. He said to me on a couple of occasions that he felt I was not pregnant (perhaps mirroring what I had felt with my previous pregnancy). I was exceptionally anxious in early pregnancy. I had continual abdominal cramping, which was quite painful, and I was sure this pregnancy too would end in miscarriage.

I really wasn't emotionally ready for the pregnancy. This time I told only my midwives that I was pregnant. We delayed telling others for a while. I read that at nine weeks pregnant you can hear the baby's heartbeat with a doppler. I had never tried to listen so early in a pregnancy before, but I thought I would try. I steeled myself in case I wasn't able to find it. It took five seconds before I found the heartbeat, regular and strong. I couldn't believe it.

It wasn't until I was fourteen weeks pregnant that I started to relax and enjoy it. I was fit and well. I resumed my exercise program, which I had slowed down in early pregnancy. In fact, I continued to do weight-training right up until just before labour started. My only concern was frequent and painful Braxton Hicks contractions that started when I was around sixteen weeks pregnant. After a while I came to realise that these were just part of the pregnancy.

Jane went into labour at 39 weeks. Her story continues in Part 3.

Janice Janice's pneumonia

At 6½ months pregnant my partner and I shifted house, and although we had plenty of help from friends and relatives I had still unintentionally overdone it. About this time I began feeling extremely tired and my bones and muscles ached.

The weeks passed and I began getting a very cold back, which I couldn't seem to warm up. As it was my first baby I didn't know what to expect and just put the whole thing down to my pregnancy. I went to the toilet one night to discover something was wrong. I just couldn't seem to sit down. I was bouncing and shaking all over, and my finger nails had gone a horrible shade of blue.

I started to panic as I began to realise something was wrong, and rang Mum, who told me to go straight to the hospital. Once at the hospital I was given an examination and told I would need my chest X-rayed. Then, to my amazement, I was told off.

'Didn't you realise something was wrong? Don't you know you could hurt the baby or damage something? You should have come to the hospital much sooner. There is nothing we can do for you at the moment. Go home, keep warm and come back in the morning for a chest X-ray. If you don't do as you are told you may end up in the hospital for a complete rest.'

Heading back home I felt amazed. I felt the telling off had been unfair, but intended doing everything I had been told. The X-ray showed I had a form of pneumonia. I had to rest for several weeks, but recovered by the time I was into the ninth month of my pregnancy.

Then, two weeks before the birth of my baby, while at a friend's place I was bitten by their dog. Shockwaves rushed through me when I couldn't pull my hand out of the dog's mouth. Eventually I managed to release my hand by forcing the dog's mouth open with my other hand. It took quite a while for the reality of what had happened to sink in. There was blood everywhere from the wound and I had a terrible feeling something bad had happened inside me.

I was still shaking, even after being cleaned up, and didn't know what to do. I was taken to the hospital for a check-up and a tetanus shot. After that I was sent home having been told everything was fine. I wasn't so sure. I almost wished I could be induced to make certain the baby was all right.

At my next check-up the doctor palpated my stomach and checked my weight gain.

'You're all baby,' he said. 'This is going to be a huge bubby – between 4 and 5 kilograms.'

The thought terrified me so much that I said to my doctor, 'Please give me a caesarean right now or let me be induced.' But my doctor wouldn't agree.

Although my baby appeared big, I hadn't gained much weight. In fact, I had lost it, and had only put on 6 kilograms my entire pregnancy. I was rather pleased about this, as I had been overweight to begin with.

Janice's birth was easier than her pregnancy. Her story is continued in Part 3.

Yvette's irritating problem

After having a fairly event-free pregnancy, in the middle of summer at around 7½ months, I went swimming, playing water volleyball with some friends. While getting dressed after the swim I noticed for the first time that I had some stretch marks on my stomach. I wondered whether they were due to my reaching and stretching for the ball in the pool.

More and more stretch marks appeared on my stomach as the pregnancy progressed. At times the stretch marks would become quite itchy and inflamed. The summer was hot and awful, and by 38 weeks I really wanted to deliver. I was having contractions irregularly, although they were not at all strong.

A few days before my due date, during my morning shower, I noticed some small, itchy red dots on one of my ankles. I thought nothing more of it, until the next morning when I noticed the rash was now quite noticeable and was also on my stretch marks, my other ankle and on the backs of my hands.

An avid needleworker, after finishing up at work I had been spending my days doing embroidery. Now that my hands were so itchy I was finding it hard to continue, as the fabric was tickling my hands and making the itching worse. Icepacks applied to the itchy places helped, but heat made things worse. The weather was so hot, which meant that at night I lay awake scratching, getting very little sleep at all. Various lotions helped, but with only limited success.

The rash continued to spread to my feet and the insides of my hands. The day before my 40-week appointment with the doctors at the hospital, I was getting desperate for some relief. I called the hospital and the midwife I spoke to suggested that I should come in to be assessed.

The doctor who assessed me prescribed a weak steroid cream (anything stronger may have harmed the baby) and ordered blood tests to see whether my liver was functioning correctly. He suggested that the only way that the rash was likely to go away would be the delivery of the baby (an option that sounded very good to me!). An internal examination revealed that all the contractions I had been having over the previous weeks had had some effect, as I was already 3 centimetres dilated. They then sent me home, with the hope that the internal exam would bring on labour. It did not.

That night I had a total of three hours sleep due to the itching. I was so fed up that I took my packed hospital bag to my doctor's appointment the next day, hoping I could convince them that they should induce me then and there. Before I could even suggest it, the obstetrician started talking about an induction due to my condition, which we eventually found out was called Pruritic Urticarial Papules and Plaques of Pregnancy (PUPPP). He booked me in for an induction the next morning. Much relieved, my husband and I went home knowing that at last the next day would be the day.

Yvette was induced the next day. Her story continues in Part 4.

Planning your baby's birth

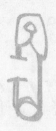

Choices, choices

Not too long ago, birth mostly took place in labour wards, with the hospital staff in total control of the labour. Fathers were not welcome at the birth. Today you can choose from several options as to how and where you would like to have your baby.

The early months of your pregnancy is the time to make plans and investigate the choices. Some women feel safer in a labour ward, others want a water birth at home. Some women wish to avoid drugs during birth, some are happy to take advantage of the available options. One of the best ways to ensure that your birth goes as you hoped is to make a birth plan, covering as many points as you think essential. Explore the alternatives available to you if your birth takes a unexpected turn – sometimes births happen so quickly there is little or no time to put the plan into place. You may want to consider the drugs available but still deliver with as little intervention as possible.

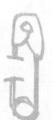

Writing your birth plan

The term 'birth plan' seems to suggest that there is some ability to control birth. In reality, this is not the case. Perhaps a better term would be 'birth preferences' or 'a wish list'. Birth plans provide a tool for letting the mother's needs be known to the health-care professional and the hospital. Birth plans often indicate that a woman wishes to avoid certain procedures or interventions, and they can help health-care professionals and support people understand more about the individual woman and her needs.

Some birth plans are very short while others are pages long. There is no correct length. It is for you to choose what issues to put in your birth plan. Some plans even include the roles of the people expected to be at the birth, such as your partner, support people and health-care professionals.

The following are some points to consider when writing a birth plan:

- choice of birthplace
- who you would like to be present at the birth
- positions during labour and birth
- mobility during labour
- music
- lighting
- clothing during labour
- photographs/video taping
- choice of pain relief strategies during labour
- medical/midwifery students
- vaginal examinations (how and when you want them)
- tears and **episiotomies**
- eating and drinking during labour
- fetal monitoring
- pushing during the **second stage** of labour
- cutting the umbilical cord
- relaxation techniques
- choices if a caesarean birth becomes necessary
- feeding the baby after the birth
- separation from baby
- choices if the baby needs to go to an intensive or special care nursery

This list is by no means exhaustive. When writing a birth plan, explore your options. Some issues will be very important to you, while other issues may not be of great concern.

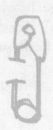

Sharing your birth plan with your midwife, obstetrician or GP

After writing a birth plan, it is helpful to discuss it with your midwife or doctor when you are around 32 to 36 weeks pregnant. This ensures that your health-care provider is fully informed of your preferences. It also permits time for either party to discuss any areas of concern and make any necessary alterations to the plan.

Some health-care practitioners do not like birth plans, as they feel they are being told what to do. Try being open: acknowledge their concerns, maintain eye contact and be assertive (not aggressive). Birth plans are ideal tools for negotiation.

Once the birth plan is finalised you can give a copy to your midwife or doctor, plus the hospital and your support people. Make sure you pack a copy of your plan in your hospital bag. Some people ask their midwife or doctor to sign their birth plan. This may make it easier for preferences to be acknowledged and followed by the hospital.

Shop around

While it is possible to come across people in the medical profession who seem to be in conflict with their patient, it should also be remembered that obstetricians and specialists are trained to save the lives of both mothers and babies. It is up to you to get to know an obstetrician's methods before you choose one for your care. Find out all you can from friends, midwives, antenatal teachers and so on. Ask the obstetrician's receptionist what percentage of patients have caesarean deliveries. If you choose an obstetrician, you will most likely be giving birth in a labour ward.

Go for your first visit with the intention of gauging the obstetrician's reactions to your questions. Be frank about what you expect. If you are not fully satisfied, you are under no obligation to visit this doctor again. This applies to birth centres and midwives. If you are unhappy with the responses to your questions or feel a lack of rapport, look for someone else.

Carol's fifth birth story

This had been my best pregnancy yet, with only one and a half months of nausea and vomiting, and then only during the first three months. I had fallen pregnant while still breastfeeding Teresa, my youngest daughter, who at the time was only nine months old. Even though I had been fairly certain of my period dates, I had been given five different due dates, but at least they were all within the same week. I had been eating really well, but had gained only 6.5 kilograms, much to my surprise.

I planned to have another hospital birth and I decided to have two support people at the birth, my friend and sister-in-law, Mary, who had been present during the births of two of my children, and my mother-in-law Laurice, who lives next door to us. My husband, Clem, was to look after our four children with the help of my brother Richard (who was staying with us).

April 18, the first due date, went by uneventfully, then so did April 20. At about 1.30 pm on April 22 I was getting regular 30-second contractions every five to ten minutes. They were not painful enough to stop me in my tracks, so I went about as usual. By 8 pm I had made a decision to go into the hospital for a check-up. I would take my packed bag with me just in case. I let Clem and Richard know what had been happening. Then I contacted Mary. I told her I would call her and Laurice to come to the hospital if necessary. Next, Clem and I headed off.

I normally have very fast one- to one-and-a-half-hour labours once my membranes have ruptured. At my 28-week check-up a **Strep B infection** had been detected, which meant that I needed an injection of antibiotics. I had to be given this injection once I was in established labour, but before the baby was born. I had been told by one of the doctors looking after me that the baby's ears, eyes or brain could be damaged during the birth or that the baby could die a few days after the birth if I didn't receive the antibiotics, so I wasn't taking any chances.

After arrival at the hospital, it was eventually established that I was in early labour. My cervix was 1 to 1.5 centimetres dilated, but my membranes couldn't be ruptured yet (to speed things up) as the baby's head was still too high. After staying in hospital for one and a half hours, nothing seemed to be happening, so I was sent back home with the words, 'You'll either be back tonight, or in the next day or two.'

Once back home, the contractions stopped altogether after having been regular for twelve hours. The contractions had not been very painful, more exciting than anything else, so it was very disappointing when they stopped. Another two days passed. It was the morning of my last due date. I wasn't expecting anything to happen, so at 3 pm the whole family went to visit a friend. I began to leak slightly, and on the way home I had my first contraction. It lasted for 45 seconds and was not too painful. It was 6.15 pm and I thought, this might be it. By the time we had reached home – several contractions and about 20 minutes later – I had made the decision to get to the hospital as soon as possible.

I called out to Laurice next door and told her we should go to the hospital right now. Then I rang Mary and told her to meet us there. I grabbed my bag and a few last-minute things, kissed Clem and the girls goodbye, then left to meet Laurice. It was the longest ten-minute drive ever, and I was so glad when we finally arrived at the hospital. Once we were there, Laurice helped me to get inside. Before I had an examination, I insisted that I be given an injection of antibiotics for the Strep B infection, as I feared the baby might be born very soon.

I was found to be 4 to 5 centimetres dilated and my cervix soft. Now that I had had the antibiotic injection, I felt relaxed and happy, and ready to give birth whenever it might happen. At 7.10 pm I got up and went to the toilet, and when I came out was relieved to see that Mary had arrived. I decided to sit rather than lie down. I requested a hot pack, which I pressed into my lower stomach area with each contraction, as the contractions had suddenly become very painful. Also, with each contraction, I looked at Mary for support (which she gave me with comforting words). The contractions were now coming every two to three minutes, lasting for one minute, and were hurting a lot.

About fifteen agonising minutes later, I got on to the bed, with a lot of help and great difficulty. I had just had a very painful long contraction, which had lasted for five minutes non-stop. Once upon the bed, I requested another examination. It was now about 7.35 pm and I was found to be 8 centimetres dilated. I had dilated 3 to 4 centimetres in only 25 minutes.

I then asked the midwife to break my membranes to speed things up. The midwife did this but there was no water left. They had indeed been leaking. The midwife commented that my membranes had been very tough.

I began to become very irritable and found it very hard not to push. Everybody (the midwives and student doctor who were present) rushed around getting ready for the baby.

I kept crying out, 'Can I push yet?'

'No, no,' was always the reply.

At 7.55 pm, I was finally allowed to push. Four minutes later, at 7.59 pm, our beautiful little boy Andrew David was born after a one-and-three-quarter-hour labour, and only 40 minutes of severe pains. We waited until the cord stopped pulsating, then Mary cut the cord.

Our little boy weighed 3335 grams, was 49 centimetres long and his **Apgar scores** at birth were 9 and then 10. I couldn't believe that Clem and I finally had a son. He did a wee on me within minutes of being born, just to show me that he was indeed a boy!

This wasn't my shortest labour so far, but it was definitely the easiest. There is absolutely nothing that can compare to the great thrill of having just given birth to a baby. Within minutes of my coming out of the delivery room, I felt I could go through another pregnancy and birth all over again.

Kuini's first birth story

When I was fifteen years old I met this wonderful woman, Joan Donaley. Joan had written the definitive book on midwifery in New Zealand. Fifteen years later I was pregnant with my first child. Delighted at being pregnant, but also a little scared of the unknown, I phoned Joan to discuss my dates and to find out when I would be due. Joan told me I was eight weeks pregnant. She checked her diary and found she was free to be my midwife, so we made an appointment to discuss the coming birth.

Joan was a wonderful, mature and secure person who had dealt with thousands of births – mostly home birthing. When we got together, we discussed my options: a home birth or a hospital birth. A little unsure, I decided on a home birth. Later, attending antenatal classes and listening to women's experiences, the women who impressed me most were those who had once or twice given birth in the hospital system, then subsequently had a home birth. These women were more zealous when discussing their stories than those who had only ever had home births. They told stories of having gone through horror and pain in the hospital system, where they were led to believe something was wrong with them and that they were poor birthers (consequently feeling very cheated), to feelings of happiness and confidence after having achieved successful births at home. This confirmed for me that I, too, was going to have a home birth.

Before the birth, my midwife visited my home three or four times, establishing a warm and trusting relationship with me. We discussed my needs, what would happen, any herbs or homoeopathic remedies I may need while I was pregnant, and also what to avoid that would hurt my baby and me. She never ever gave me an internal examination during this period. According to Joan, to be eligible for a home birth you must not smoke and you must eat a balanced diet. I felt very healthy and happy.

Kuini had a home birth as planned. Her story continues in Part 3.

Preparing to be both stubborn and flexible

Birth plans should be written in a way that allows flexibility. It really is impossible to account for every variation of labour on a birth plan, and it may not be possible to follow your plan if something unpredictable occurs. When writing your birth plan it is better to use words like 'I would prefer' or 'if possible'. This helps prevent the birth plan being seen as inflexible or as a list of dos and don'ts that must be followed. Birth plans simply indicate the preferences of the woman in labour and provide an outline of how she would like the birth to be.

On the other hand, you may be faced with a health-care provider unhappy with your decisions. In an ideal world it would be great to be able to negotiate a mutually acceptable outcome. However, this may not always be possible. In some instances a woman may decide to take a stand against some procedure or intervention. The assistance of the woman's partner and/or support people is very important, as they may be called upon to advocate for her. Remember, you have a right to refuse any procedure. Every procedure carried out must have the woman's consent. A procedure carried out without consent is considered to be assault.

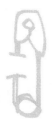

Deciding for yourself

As situations arise during your pregnancy or labour you may be presented with options or suggestions for drugs or other medical intervention. Sometimes there is no choice. Other times, however, there is often an alternative course of action. It can be difficult to decide which is the right way to go. Finding out as much as you can beforehand is one way to gain confidence. The following steps may help you with your decision:

1 Identify the issue/problem.
2 Identify what the desired outcome is.
3 Think about what is needed to achieve the desired outcome. It is helpful to gather information from the following sources: personal knowledge, health-care professionals, family, friends, books, the internet.
4 Explore the alternatives. Think about what result the alternatives may have. Are there risks? What are the emotional implications of the alternative courses of action?
5 Make the decision.
6 Carry out the decision.
7 Evaluate the decision.

This process is ideal for working through any problems that may arise during the pregnancy, birth or afterwards. Obviously, the more time there is available, the more informed the decision. If it is an emergency situation, there may be little time for gathering information from alternative sources. In this case there is little choice but to place trust with the health-care professional. Being prepared beforehand is always useful. For instance, you may want a drug-free delivery, but knowing about **epidurals** and their effects can be helpful should you be advised to have an epidural by medical staff. Or if you would like to give birth at a birth centre, but discover you have a condition that requires a labour ward, having a Plan B worked out may help you make the final decision and know more fully what you want from that labour-ward birth.

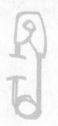

Planning where and how to have your baby

Whether you write a birth plan or not, you will have to make a decision about where to give birth to your child. The following alternatives and stories may help you make up your mind.

Birth centre

A birth centre is normally run by midwives, who look after you throughout your pregnancy as well as for the delivery of your child. Active **natural birthing** is encouraged, with emphasis on a drug-free labour. Natural pain-relieving methods, such as upright positions – for example, leaning against furniture, sitting upright, walking around, leaning into a beanbag – and the use of **birth stools** are encouraged. Hot-water showers, spas and hot packs are also utilised.

Family and friends who will support you rather than simply witness the birth are encouraged to attend. Children are also welcome if they are accompanied by their own support adult.

Care is taken to create a natural environment, with the option of dimmed lighting and your own music being played. The birth centre sets out to create a comfortable, homely atmosphere where you will be attended by registered midwives who, in many cases, will be backed by the full medical profession, if needed, especially if the centre is attached to a maternity hospital.

In most cases, the baby's umbilical cord is not clamped and cut until the cord has stopped pulsating. Breastfeeding following delivery is encouraged to facilitate the natural delivery of the placenta without the routine use of the drug **Syntocinon** to speed things up.

Midwives in the birth centre try to be as unobtrusive as possible, preferring to use less invasive measures to monitor progress. For example, a trumpet may be used instead of a heart monitor. They also try to avoid the use of drugs such as **pethidine** and gas.

Inductions, epidurals and caesareans are not carried out in the birth centre, but the woman can and will be transferred if these procedures become necessary. It is also standard policy to transfer women if **meconium** is present in the waters.

A birth centre is a popular place to give birth, so you will probably need to book in early. Your first appointment will be around ten to twelve weeks, with monthly check-ups until 28 weeks, fortnightly visits until 36 weeks, and thereafter weekly appointments.

A doctor will offer you a health check and assess your eligibility to give birth in the birth centre. The usual pregnancy tests are offered through the centre. Blood tests to check for spina bifida, Down's syndrome and other abnormalities will be offered, as well as an ultrasound at about eighteen weeks.

On your first visit, you will have blood drawn to check for blood type, immunity to infectious diseases, haemoglobin level and so on. Your due date will be worked out, your history taken and you will be booked in to have your baby. You will also be given a routine check-up.

Your subsequent antenatal appointments will include blood pressure being taken, a sample of your urine tested, the baby's heartbeat listened to and your fundal height checked. You will also be given the opportunity to discuss any worries you might have. At later visits, you may also be screened for gestational diabetes and the Strep B infection.

At most birth centres, plenty of reading material is available. Photograph albums showing women delivering their babies are also usual.

As long as you ask permission, you can also arrange for photographs and videos to be taken – professional or otherwise.

Once your baby is born, after initially being held and nursed by you, he or she will then be checked by the midwife and weighed and measured. A crib with blankets will be provided.

Your baby will also be checked by a paediatrician before you go home, and you will be examined too. If all is well you may even go home within hours of your delivery or on the same day. However, if you wish, you could also be transferred to the postnatal wards, where you can stay until you are ready to leave (normally four days).

If you take advantage of the early home discharge program, a midwife will come to your home over the next week to check on you and your baby.

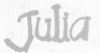

Julia's birth story

Julia's story continues from Part 1. She had been admitted to hospital with high blood pressure but had been allowed home. She wanted to give birth in a birth centre.

I awoke to a dull ache not unlike a period cramp. I secretly thought my labour might be starting, but wanted to keep it to myself just in case it wasn't. This dull, achy pain turned out to be continual, but didn't worry me. Later that day, my farewell party was being held at work. I didn't say anything to anyone about how I was feeling, but laughed when someone commented on how pale I looked. 'I feel fine,' I said.

That night when I went to the toilet, I noticed a big, bloody show. That evening I found it hard to sleep (more from excitement than anything else). I filled myself a hot-water bottle to help with the pain. It wasn't until 10 am the next day that things really became uncomfortable. Now the pain was more intense and coming between breaks, although still manageable. My mum is not alive and it was during this time that a friend's mum phoned to see if I'd had my baby yet. I told her what was happening and began asking her lots of questions. She was a big help, giving me all the answers I needed.

Once off the phone, I began crouching forward onto the lounge to alleviate the pains. After four hours of this, I then made my first call to the birth centre. They told me this was pre-labour and that these weren't contractions, as I sounded 'too well' to be having them. 'Oh no,' I thought, 'what is true labour going to be like then?'

By late afternoon I got myself into the bath, which worked like a dream. It was just amazing how it eased the pain. I lay there for the next three hours, occasionally adding hot water. By early evening I was starting to feel ill and at 7 pm I vomited. This really disturbed me, so I rang the birth centre a second time, but now became frustrated with what they told me. 'The contractions don't sound like labour, and the vomiting is nothing to worry about.'

However, the midwife did tell me to come straight in if I started feeling too uncomfortable, or was worried about being at home. By this stage, the pains were very close together, coming every three minutes, and my husband, John, was starting to become worried by my obvious pain. But I trusted what the midwife had told me, and wondered how much worse these pains were going to get.

Two hours later, I rang the birth centre after vomiting once again. It was decided that if I vomited yet again, I would go in.

Things were becoming unbearable. One hour later, after being sick a third time, I rang the birth centre saying, 'We're on our way.' Once we arrived, I vomited just outside the birth centre. Helen, the midwife, was waiting for us at the front door. It was such a relief to see her there. But she waited one whole hour before she examined me. The examination hurt a lot. Then Helen told me the bad news. I was only 1 centimetre dilated. 'Oh no,' I thought. 'How am I going to get through this?'

I found that walking really helped. I must have walked 10 kilometres. After a couple of hours, Helen came back and asked if I was okay, suggesting I try the shower. She was right. It did ease the pain, and I stayed in there for the next two hours. Then, at about 5 am, Helen came back and told me she wanted to do another examination. Remembering the last one, I asked if it could wait for another hour or so. I couldn't bear to get out of the shower, so Helen agreed to wait until 6 am. In the meantime, I believed another hour should lead to another 2 centimetres or more of **dilation**.

How wrong I proved to be! During the examination, Helen discovered I was only 3 centimetres dilated. I couldn't believe it. How could all this pain have achieved so little? Helen also told me she had noticed meconium and that I would have to be transferred to the labour ward. [This is a requirement of birth centres.]

I didn't want to go there, so asked if I could spend some time in the therapeutic bath. Someone had told me about this bath being able to speed up your labour, and I was hoping for a miracle. I desperately wanted this to be a natural birth, but knew if I was sent up to the labour ward I wouldn't be able to bear the pain any more and would end up having an epidural. This would mean all that work for nothing. For me, it was important to be able to cope without drugs and, to my relief, Helen did let me get into the bath.

It was boiling. I began to panic, wondering what was going to happen next. Then, about five minutes later, this huge blob of bloody material came out of me. This upset my husband but Helen said, 'That's great. This means your labour is progressing well and your cervix is softening up.' I didn't care. It was just so hot.

Ten minutes later, I felt a desperate urge to open my bowels. Helen said, 'That's wonderful. It's the baby's head coming.' I couldn't believe it.

It was now 6.30 am and I was asked to get out of the bath. Another midwife, Sheryl, had started her shift. I told them I didn't want to go to the labour ward and didn't think I could make it there anyway. They then rang the obstetrician, telling him about the meconium. In the meantime, I made my way over to the beanbag, which had been lined with plastic ready for the birth.

Once I reached it, I began pushing. It was such an exhilarating experience and not the agony I had imagined. In fact, I couldn't get enough of it. I pushed for the next 40 minutes with every contraction that came. They were now coming every two minutes and lasting for 60 seconds. Then Sheryl noticed the baby's head **crowning** and told me to stop pushing and to pant instead.

I was leaning on all fours over the beanbag and making an involuntary primitive grunting sound. After about five minutes of panting, Helen and Sheryl now told me, 'The head's not disappearing any more. It won't be long,' and I was told to start pushing again. Sheryl was supporting my **perineum** as well as the baby's head, and was massaging the baby as it came through. Two more pushes and the baby completely emerged.

It was finally out. 'I've done it,' was my first thought. 'I've given birth!'

Sheryl and Helen suctioned our baby just as a precautionary measure because of the meconium she had passed. Then she was shown to John, who immediately wanted me to see our baby also.

'It's little Ursula,' I said as soon as I saw her. All through my pregnancy I had thought I was having a boy, but seeing a girl, the name sprang into my mind. She was taken away to be checked, weighed and measured. Ursula was born at 7.27 am, weighing 3040 grams and measuring 52 centimetres.

About twenty minutes after our baby's birth, the placenta came out. I don't remember much else, except I now had a daughter and was on such an incredible high. I felt euphoric.

Meconium

Meconium is a tar-like, dark substance that is the baby's first bowel motion. Sometimes babies pass this meconium into the **amniotic fluid** before they are born. When the water around the baby is stained with thick meconium, there is an increased risk of complications for the baby. If the meconium staining is only light, there is dispute as to whether there is any need for concern at all. Babies who experience a lack of oxygen may pass meconium into the amniotic fluid. However, babies who are well may also pass meconium into the waters. One reason they may do this is because they are mature. Careful monitoring is carried out during labour to identify any babies who may be experiencing distress.

Jesenka's birth story

Jesenka's story continues from Part 1. She was keen to have a natural birth at a birth centre.

On Tuesday 16 August, after I had my ultrasound, my husband, Phillip, and I were picking up our daughter, Merita, from school when my contractions began. They were quite strong (in fact, I had to stop walking while I had one) and were twenty minutes apart. Then, while we were doing some shopping, they became even stronger. At 5.30 pm I rang the birth centre and was told to wait until the pains were five minutes apart, lasting one minute, and then to wait another hour before I came in. I had just put the phone down when the pains did start corning every five minutes, being so strong I had to stop everything. But I did find relief standing and hanging from Phillip's neck while he massaged my lower back.

Twenty minutes later, the pains were coming three to five minutes apart. I rang back the birth centre and the midwife told me to come straight in. By the time we arrived at the hospital shortly before 7 pm, I was heavily in labour. Going straight to the birth suite, I lay on the bed, feeling most comfortable on my side.

Phillip now massaged my lower back, which gave me some relief, and I also used the hot pack, which helped. After a while I thought a hot shower would ease the pain, but it didn't so I soon got out. I went to the edge of the bed feeling like I was going to be sick, and I was. Afterwards, I actually felt better. Phillip rubbed my back again, which also helped me feel better.

I wanted to use the toilet, but couldn't. The midwife told me what I was feeling was pressure from the baby's head and helped me off the toilet. I went to the side of the bed feeling an urge to squat, but my legs were so weak that I found myself sinking to the floor. A mat was pulled out for me and I was helped onto it. Soon I asked for a beanbag, which I practically lay on. The pain was getting so strong that I asked for the gas. The midwife said I could have it, but Phillip was trying to persuade me not to. Each time the pains stopped I felt fine, but during the contractions the pain was so unbearable I just couldn't stand it.

'It hurts and I want the gas. I want the pains to go away,' I kept saying. I felt confused because I'd been told I could have the gas, but no one was bringing it to me. So instead I gained relief by squeezing Phillip's hand very, very hard. He later told me I nearly broke his fingers.

While I was in this position on the beanbag, and pushing and screaming from pain, my father and daughter came in. Thinking all this groaning and screaming would scare my daughter, I told them to leave. Not long after they had left, I began to start pushing. I needed to be upright, so was helped into a kneeling position, supporting myself with my hands around my husband's neck. The pains at this stage were very, very strong, but not lasting very long.

Just before the baby started coming out, I felt a great gush of water and some very strong pain. I was groaning and crying because the baby's head felt so huge. The head started to come out and I was told to stop pushing. When I started pushing again, the baby's shoulders started coming and it felt very big. At one time while I was pushing, I felt myself sinking into the ground, so needed to be pushed back up again. After my baby's shoulders were out, I pushed a few more times until our baby was completely out.

Phillip was sitting in front of me and saw our baby being born, so straight away cried, 'It's a boy!' But because I was so dazed from the pain, I didn't hear him. So with my baby between my legs, I leaned into the beanbag while the midwife helped me straighten myself. Then I picked up our baby to look at him.

I found I had given birth to a son and was absolutely thrilled. It was 8.30 pm. I placed a towel over our baby (one I had brought from home), then immediately put him to my breast, but he wouldn't start sucking. Shortly after this my daughter and father came back into the room. A couple of minutes after they arrived, the placenta popped straight out, even though it was still attached to our baby. The cord was not pulsating, so it was clamped and Phillip cut it.

I held our baby facing my husband and said, 'What do you think?' Meaning, what shall we call him? Phillip understood what I meant, and said, 'Matthew.' As Phillip and I had already discussed names for our baby while I had been pregnant, we agreed straight away. It pleased me that such a nice name suited our baby so well.

I looked down at Matthew to discover he had done a poo on me. The midwife cleaned him up, then also helped me clean myself. She then weighed and dressed Matthew before giving him back to me, telling me his weight was 3464 grams. Our baby's Apgar scores after he was born were 9 at one minute, then 10 at five minutes.

From the time of our baby's delivery until now, the lights had been kept dimmed so we could shield his eyes. (I had done this so his eyes could gradually adjust.)

Immediately following his birth, Matthew had given a couple of cries but had stopped crying when I picked him up. I was surprised at how inquisitive and active he was, preferring to look around than feed. Phillip and Dad now wanted to hold Matthew, so I took this opportunity to shower and get dressed. By 10 pm Matthew finally felt hungry, so I put him to my breast and fed him for half an hour. Photographs were also taken.

Matthew and I were both well, so I was given the option to go up to the postnatal ward for a few days or go home. I decided to go home, as I felt I could better relax there. We were discharged at 12.30 pm, only four hours after I had given birth.

Labour ward

Labour wards contain all the facilities needed for childbirth, and have the ability to deal with complications should they arise. Blood tests, **electronic fetal heart monitoring**, epidurals and other forms of pain relief can all be quickly provided. Many hospitals today are more sympathetic than they were in the past to women giving birth. Fathers and other support people are welcome at the birth and able to be involved where appropriate.

It is wise to understand that a labour ward is part of a hospital and is run accordingly. Staff work in shifts, and it is likely that there will be at least one staff change while you are in labour. This means that you and the new staff will have to catch up with each other. Midwives are very experienced and it does not take long for them to familiarise themselves with your stage of birth and requirements. Keep your birth plan handy if you have specific wishes.

In a labour ward you are more likely to be encouraged to use pain relief, or possibly pressured into procedures you may wish to avoid. Some doctors still perform episiotomies as a standard practice. Hospitals can be more concerned with time and efficiency than the requirements of a natural birth. In the event of a labour that is progressing slowly, there can be pressure on you to induce the birth or, after the birth, have Syntocinon to hasten the birth of the placenta. You may be happy to accept any of these procedures, and it is good to know they are an available option. It may be that you request such options even before they are offered. You may, however, wish to wait before having a procedure, or decline it all together. This may require you to be firm, and support people can be a boon in these circumstances. In any case, if you understand the hospital system you are less likely to be distressed or dismayed at what may occur. For many, the knowledge that everything is on hand in case of complications is worth foregoing some of their wishes for the birth plan.

Find out as much as you can about your hospital before you make your final choice. In Australia, it is mandatory for hospitals to provide statistics on obstetric interventions to the Department of Health. Regrettably, this information is not always easy to access. In New South Wales the information is publicly available on the internet. However, it is not so easy in other states. Ask staff, other mothers and midwives about the level of intervention and the hospital's attitudes towards birth. For instance, some have much higher rates of caesarean sections than do others.

If you are choosing a labour ward the attitude of your doctor is quite important. Where the doctor is responsible for your care, the midwives are required to follow his or her instructions regarding the birth. Work out what is important for you and make sure you and your obstetrician are on the same wavelength. If you have strong feelings about the birth, as mentioned earlier in this section, write a birth plan and show it to your doctor and the staff so that everyone is comfortable with what you want. Also, remember to be flexible. Hospital staff are dedicated to the health of the mother and baby and wish to achieve this within the context of their knowledge. There are some bleak stories of hospital births, but many of the staff will be as helpful to you as possible.

Remember, too, that you may not be the only one giving birth and the staff may need to accommodate a variety of situations and labours. If you are fortunate, it will be a quiet time in the labour ward when you go in. During a recent busy time at a maternity hospital, one of the fathers fainted, blocking shut the door into the birth suite. It took two nurses to push the door open and then attend to the prone father and the labouring and anxious mother.

Once your pregnancy is confirmed and you have decided on your doctor (or midwife) and hospital, you need to contact the hospital and book in for your birth. Speak to the booking administrator at the hospital. On your visit to book in, you will be shown around the labour ward and told about antenatal classes and their cost. Most large maternity hospitals have comfortable birth rooms or suites, and providing there are no problems with the birth, you will give birth in this room. However, if the labour slows down or stops, you may be asked to either return home or go to a waiting room, as beds can sometimes be at a premium.

Prepare your labour kit in advance and include some personal things to make you feel more relaxed (though nothing that you would not like to lose). Having support people in hospital will sustain you and give you backup if choices need to be made during the birth. In some hospitals you can have your own midwife at the hospital; at others she can be there as a support person only.

Depending on your labour, your hospital stay can be quite short. Some women opt to go home within hours of giving birth. First-time mothers often prefer to stay until they feel more assured and the baby is breastfeeding easily (see Part 6). Mothers with several children can welcome the rest! Unless there are medical reasons, the usual stay is no longer than four days after the birth.

Donna's first
birth story

Donna had experienced swelling and high blood pressure in pregnancy. Her story continues from Part 1.

Steve, my husband, was supposed to pick me up after my check-up, but we somehow managed to miss each other and I now had to catch the bus home. Then it happened. I began experiencing shooting pains travelling all the way from my pubic bone to my stomach. I thought it was because I had done too much walking, but then realised that they were regular pains. I must have experienced four pains during that twenty-minute bus trip and was very embarrassed, desperately hoping no one was noticing me jumping off my seat. I now became angry with Steve, as I wouldn't have been going through this bad experience if he had picked me up as he said he would.

It is a ten-minute walk from the bus stop to our place, but it took me half an hour because the pains made me walk so slowly. When I did finally reach home, I thought that maybe all this had happened because my bladder was over-full. Maybe if I went to the toilet it would relieve the pain, I thought, but I sat there for about twenty minutes unable to do anything. Then it dawned on me that my labour might be starting. When Steve finally returned home, we both said, 'Where were you?' Then I told him how long I had been sitting on the toilet unable to relieve the pressure.

One hour later, at 5 pm, I noticed the pains again. Realising that they were coming every five minutes, I decided to ring Mum to check if she thought they were contractions. I didn't want to ring the hospital in case it was a false alarm, as I still felt there was a chance this was due to overexertion, but Mum assured me I was in labour.

I rang the hospital and was told to wait for about two hours, until the contractions were two minutes apart, before coming in. I wasn't long off the phone when my brother and his friend arrived. When my brother noticed I was having regular pains, he told me not to wait but to go straight to the hospital. As it turned out, this was very good advice. The trip to the hospital was quite an experience because Steve was driving like a maniac. It was not that he was driving fast, but he was driving through red lights and constantly asking me, 'Are you all right? You're not going to have the baby now, are you?'

Somehow we arrived safely at the hospital and the midwife gave me a check-up. I asked how long it would be before the baby was born, to which she replied, 'Relax for a while – have a shower and the baby should be born by 3 am tomorrow.' As it was still only 7 pm, I hoped she was wrong and that it would be a lot earlier.

Some time later my uncle appeared. 'A drink would be nice,' I told him. But, by the time he returned, I no longer felt like a drink and wasn't comprehending who was there and what was going on. (I was on some sort of natural high.) My contractions were now two minutes apart and I was standing up pushing into the rail with each one. Not long afterwards I walked back to the labour ward. The midwife checked me again, saying, 'Oh my, you're already 8 centimetres dilated!' Now I knew why I was experiencing such strong pains.

Soon after my examination, my contractions seemed to get even stronger. I got into the shower but was unable to relieve the pain. I didn't know whether to sit or stand, as every position was uncomfortable. Then, after my shower, the midwife made me lie down so the monitors could be placed across my stomach. My pains now became almost unbearable. They had a monitor checking me and another one checking the baby because my contractions were coming so quickly. I asked the nurse what they were monitoring for, only to be told that they had lost the baby's heartbeat. That was, to say the least, upsetting. Steve and I just looked at each other hoping everything was okay.

It was now 10.30 pm. My waters still hadn't broken, so the midwife ruptured them, telling me it shouldn't be long now. Soon after that I remember being told it was time to push, which was great considering I was already feeling the urge. I now thought to myself, the harder and stronger I push, the quicker I can get this over and done with. Steve gave me some crushed ice and was wiping my forehead, as I was starting to sweat. It was a good feeling to know he was there. I was offered the gas mask, but because I couldn't stand the thought of covering my face I preferred to take nothing at all. Then suddenly the baby's head was starting to show.

'I can see its hair,' Steve said. 'It's about as big as a twenty-cent piece.' Both he and the midwife now said, 'Come on, push, push.' But each time I did, I felt like my face would explode. Then when the contraction stopped I would actually doze off to sleep. But these little naps gave me the energy I needed to continue pushing. Then it finally happened. The baby's head came out completely. 'The head is through – don't push,' I heard someone say. I felt ecstatic.

Once given the go-ahead, I quickly pushed the rest of our baby out. 'It's a boy!' was the first thing I heard an excited Steve say. Soon after our baby was born, his cord was cut and he was taken away to be checked. Meanwhile, my legs began to shake uncontrollably and Steve and I were both wondering what was going on. We assumed this must be normal when it did later stop.

I was soon congratulated and given a cup of tea. I didn't know what to feel. I had just had a baby, but I was shaking uncontrollably, and where was my baby? He was finally brought back, but I still felt blank. It wasn't until I had a chance to let what had happened sink in that I began to feel excited. I couldn't get to sleep, even though it was late and I was tired. I was on such a high and just couldn't stop looking at my baby. It was definitely the most wonderful and incredible experience.

Home birth

Childbirth at home can be a special family event. Home birth provides continuity of care with a midwife who comes to know the whole family. Your midwife will ensure the pregnancy is remaining healthy and that the baby's development is normal. Being able to choose your own caregiver who will attend throughout the birth is very reassuring to the mother, father and support people. Siblings enjoy mum not having to leave the home. Knowing she can call her midwife when the time is right makes the woman feel more relaxed, and this facilitates an easier birth. At home you are free to move around, occupying yourself as you please until the contractions become too painful. At home there are activities and distractions that aid an active birth, from doing the vacuuming to walking in the garden.

Preparing for a home birth is an enjoyable experience. You may already have a midwife in mind, but if you haven't, ask friends and/or contact the various midwife associations for recommendations. Talk to the midwife to see if you have the same beliefs and approach to childbirth. Once you have made your choice, you can discuss your plans at length during antenatal visits. The midwife will provide a list of things your will need to get ready. This is not a major affair. In fact, mothers mostly enjoy getting ready for a home birth.

There are few requirements. One usual article is some form of protective floor covering, such as a plastic sheet covered by some old bedsheets. The mother or midwife can provide this. Your home does not need to be sterile, nor do towels, blankets and other things for the baby. However, everything does need to be clean, with towels and so on washed and stored in a clean cupboard. During the pregnancy, the midwife will visit the home to familiarise herself with the layout and facilities. There is plenty of time to discuss individual needs.

Only women with low-risk pregnancies are suitable for a home birth (this means where there are no major health problems with the mother or baby and the pregnancy has continued normally). Unfortunately, sometimes mothers and babies are unwell. Where there is an identified high-risk birth, such as women with pre-eclampsia, diabetes, any bleeding in the second half of pregnancy, a growth-restricted baby, and placenta praevia, the medical support provided in a hospital labour ward is essential. For women with twins or a breech birth, it is generally considered safer to be in hospital. Some women and their partners still prefer to be at home and will engage two experienced midwives for their birth, increasing the safety.

It can be reassuring to know where the nearest maternity hospital is and to have made some contact with the staff. Some hospitals are more responsive than others to mothers planning a home birth.

The freedom of movement, the comfort of familiar surroundings and the continuity of care can make birth at home a relaxing and rewarding experience.

Carol's seventh birth story

Carol

Thirty-eight weeks pregnant, sick and tired of everything, I hoped this baby might come a little early. Considering that my six previous children had mostly come before or on their due dates, I thought this was likely. I had gained only 8.5 kilograms, but nevertheless still felt large and uncomfortable. With previous pregnancies, I had always experienced Braxton Hicks pains for up to six weeks before delivery, but with this baby I had not even felt one. Maybe this was a sign that the baby would be overdue.

So when, on a Wednesday night, at 38½ weeks, my contractions started, I immediately began timing them. I soon became disappointed when I realised they were not painful, and only lasting for 45 seconds. One hour later they stopped altogether. I must have known it was not the real thing, for I didn't phone the midwife, or my support people, even though I was having a home birth and my labours normally last only one to one and a half hours.

Five days later, my 39-week check-up showed my blood pressure still perfect, 120/70. The midwife, Cathy, commented that she could no longer feel the baby's head, meaning that the baby had descended and labour could start at any time. All week I had been having shows. August 12 was my due date. Desperate to start labour, I went for a fast walk to the corner store. I did experience a couple of pains during that walk, but nothing when I got back home. By 10 pm, however, I recognised the signs of imminent labour – a weird feeling and a glassy look in my eyes. 'I'll be waking up in labour,' I told Clem and myself before I went to bed.

Sure enough, at 1.45 am I was brought out of my sleep by a strong pain. Fearing a quick birth, I charged out of bed, stopping only to time the contractions before phoning my midwife. My contractions were coming every three minutes, lasting 45 seconds. I ignored the fact that they weren't really painful, but insisted Cathy should come straight away in case of a quick labour. Next I rang my support person, Mary, and the photographer, Nicole, who is also a midwife. My contractions continued to last for 45 seconds, coming every three to six minutes. So, at 3.30 am, Cathy gave me my first examination and discovered I was 4 to 5 centimetres dilated.

Being at home was wonderful. I had a shower when I felt like it and walked around and tidied up. I did all of this while experiencing contractions, and my contractions never felt more than mild. In fact, because of this I was never convinced that I was dilating, so when, several hours later, Cathy found that I was 8 centimetres dilated, I couldn't believe it. I sat down to chat with Mary, then the pain hit me, so I immediately stood up again. As it turned out, my contractions weren't painful as long as I stood, but did, however, become painful when I sat or lay down.

By 8 am, all the children were awake. Cathy gave me a third examination and declared me fully dilated and ready to push the baby out. 'But I'm not feeling like pushing,' I told her. 'I can hardly believe I'm 10 centimetres dilated. My contractions haven't felt stronger than Braxton Hicks.'

I knew everyone was expecting me to give birth, but I just didn't want to with so many people around. So instead I ran around getting everyone dressed and ready for school. For the next hour, I completely forgot I was having a baby. I did up zippers, put on shoes and combed hair. My contractions continued to be only mild.

Finally, at 9 am, Mary said to me, 'Everyone's gone now. You can have the baby.' Obligingly, I entered my bedroom, but I still didn't feel like pushing. I simply didn't have any urges to do so. Over the next hour, I half-heartedly pushed with every contraction that came, trying out different positions in the process. I lay down, stood up, squatted and leaned over the furniture, but eventually settled on the bed. I lay on my back and Mary and Cathy took charge. Each woman held one of my hands and instructed me to push. 'Push, push. Keep going,' I was told with every contraction. I was also given a mirror to encourage me, which it did once I saw the dark hair emerging.

At 10.10 am, after an eight-and-a-half-hour labour (my longest yet), our baby was finally born. It was a boy! I could hardly believe how elated I felt. I had actually enjoyed the labour and here I was holding my longed-for baby – a second son for Clem and me.

I have never felt so happy in my whole life as when I gave birth to James. I accredit my almost painless labour to the fact that I had a home birth. I had been completely uninhibited and had done as I pleased throughout my entire labour.

This labour was very different from my hospital birth with my first-born, Amanda. During that 3½-hour drug-managed labour, I was knocked out with pethidine, which made me disoriented and distressed during contractions, screaming through every one. Amanda's birth weight had been 2715 grams and James's birth weight 3300 grams, so obviously size had nothing to do with it.

I hadn't avoided pain during second stage labour with James, but this only added to the satisfaction and sense of achievement I felt afterwards.

Active birth

Janet Balaskas, the founder of the Active Birth Movement, was the first to use the term 'active birth'. The term came about to counter the medical term 'active management of birth', which medicalises birth by placing time limits on the length of labour and involves the liberal use of the drug Syntocinon to speed up labour. The philosophy behind active birth is that the majority of labours will progress without complications when they are not hindered by routine interventions. Active birth is about being able to give birth naturally, where a woman follows her instincts and trusts in the natural process. Active birth is also about being upright and using physiologically ideal positions during the labour and birth. In an active birth, women move about freely during the labour.

There are many advantages to active birth. Being upright and active can help shorten the length of labour. Upright, active positions during the **first stage of labour** include walking, standing, squatting, sitting and kneeling. The use of active birth positions during the second stage of labour makes optimum use of gravity to facilitate the descent of the baby down the birth canal. These positions can actually enlarge the outlet of the pelvis, thus making the passage of the baby easier. Active birth positions in the second stage of labour include standing, a standing squat, the supported squat and kneeling. Women also use the hands and knees (all-fours) position, as it allows the pelvis to open to its widest capacity. However, it has a drawback of not utilising the aid of gravity.

Active birth aims to empower women to give birth under their own steam, without medical interference, and helps women experience a positive start to parenthood.

Laura's birth story

I was sick from the first week of my pregnancy, even before I found out that I was pregnant. Once certain, I looked into nutrition and vitamin supplements and began eating completely natural foods, as I found this calmed my nausea. Even so, the morning sickness persisted until I was three months pregnant, as did my feeling of extreme fatigue.

The rest of my pregnancy was fairly uneventful, apart from my stomach, which was huge throughout. From three months on I was full of energy and continued my normal routine of exercising, cycling and swimming, although I did take it easier than I normally do. I was also doing antenatal yoga in preparation for the delivery.

Once I knew I was pregnant, I booked myself into the birth centre and employed a midwife named Julie. Throughout my pregnancy, Julie came to my home, where she did all my antenatal examinations. By the time I was due to have the baby, Julie and I had developed a strong friendship and she understood what I wanted for the birth.

Three days before my due date, my waters broke. Because Julie was a private midwife she was prepared to let me go into labour naturally rather than induce the baby, but unfortunately two days later my labour had still not started. Julie now decided that I needed to be induced, so had me attend the birth centre, where she set up a Syntocinon drip to get my contractions going. At the time, I wasn't very pleased, as I had planned a completely natural birth.

Within half an hour of the drip being started I was experiencing strong contractions every ten minutes, so I spent half an hour in the shower, drip and all, trying to ease the pain. I became a little anxious while standing in the shower, as my legs were shaking and I was a bit shocked at the strength of the contractions. I had not expected labour to be quite so painful.

With my drip still attached, I got out of the shower and into a hot bath. Bradley, my partner, ran really hot water over my stomach with the shower connection. I also had a lit candle next to the bath, as well as music gently playing. Julie was saying encouraging, positive things that I found really helpful. Eventually, I reached the stage where I couldn't stand lying back in the bath anymore. I got onto my hands and knees while still in the bath. I spent four hours in there until I couldn't handle the heat any longer. Throughout the time I was in the bath, Bradley massaged my back and stomach whenever I had a contraction.

Because I was so hot, Julie suggested I might feel better on the bed, so I spent a fair bit of time on the bed on my hands and knees. Julie was bringing me hot packs for my stomach and back, which were wonderful, but the contractions were still painful. By this stage, they were very close together and all I wanted was to go home and go to bed. There was just no time for me to rest between them. In my mind, I thought I was screaming and yelling, but apparently I wasn't. I felt as though I was trapped inside a body that was out of control and remember thinking that the pain was going to go on forever with no escape. I actually resigned myself to this, but later found out I must have been in **transition**.

I found second stage a lot easier than first, as I now had some control over what was happening and could actually do something active. I stood up and pushed, but wasn't getting very far, so Julie suggested kneeling might be better.

Now kneeling with my arms around Bradley's waist while he sat on the bed, I found it helpful having Bradley next to my face. I remember at one point asking, 'Is the head out yet?' to which Julie replied, 'I can't even see it.' I just couldn't believe it. The whole experience seemed totally divorced from the fact that I was having a baby. All I was concerned about was getting rid of this pain. I couldn't believe that my body still had to stretch further than it already had. Julie was putting hot packs and applying some oil onto my perineum, which felt lovely. I'm sure her doing this is what saved me from tearing and needing stitches.

Finally the head came out and Julie asked if I wanted to feel it. At that time, I didn't really care, but felt it anyway. Then one more push and our baby was out.

At this point, the pain completely disappeared. So, on top of the relief of having no more pain, I was now holding this gorgeous, most exquisite child, screaming with laughter, joy and happiness. It was an amazing experience. Our baby was a girl and we were stunned at how perfect she was. We couldn't take our eyes off her.

The third-stage delivery of my placenta was almost a non-event. One push and it was over.

Our baby weighed 3850 grams and was 51 centimetres long, being born after an eight-hour labour. I felt really strong and proud of myself for achieving the natural labour I wanted.

Water birth

The use of water has become increasingly popular as a way of avoiding a high-tech birth both in hospital and at home. The use of water during labour is well-accepted and quite commonplace. However, giving birth to a baby under water is more controversial and many questions arise when a woman considers giving birth this way. Is water birth safe? Are there any benefits of water birth? What steps should women follow if they wish to use water during labour and birth? Water birth is currently in need of extensive research. Some evidence from around the world on water births is being gathered, and hopefully in the future we will know a lot more. For now we have to use the limited evidence available.

The use of water during labour is very popular with women. The majority of women who use warm showers, baths or theraputic spas during labour (but not necessarily for the birth) say that they would use water again in their next labour. The many perceived benefits of water include: reduced pain, greater mobility due to buoyancy, and a greater ability to relax. The use of water may also reduce tears to the perineum, and it is a gentle entrance into the world for the baby.

Some people fear that the baby will drown if born into water. The current evidence suggests that this does not occur. Babies have what is called a diving reflex that helps prevent them breathing water into their lungs. When a baby is brought to the surface of the water, the cool air touches the receptors present on the baby's face and trigger the baby to begin breathing.

There are essential steps recommended when planning a water birth. Some of these steps include ensuring that:

◊ a skilled health-care practitioner in water birth is available

◊ a normal labour and birth is expected

◊ the pool or bath has been thoroughly cleaned

◊ the water is not too hot (less than 36°C)

◊ no additives are put in the water

◊ the baby's face is brought to the surface of the water as soon as it is born.

Arranging the use of water during labour is often easy. Many hospitals and birth centres have baths and sometimes pools available. However, the possibility for a full water birth within hospitals depends very much on the skills of the staff and on hospital policies. Women exploring the option of water birth need to contact their local maternity hospital to find out more. Arranging a water birth at home is usually easy. Most home-birth midwives are skilled at water birth and will advise on organising a suitable pool and the equipment needed.

Cathy's water birth

Having a baby and becoming a mother is something I had wanted since I was twelve years old. Now, finally, eighteen years later, my dream had come true. The pregnancy wasn't as easygoing as I thought it would be, mainly as a result of my being very emotional. Nigel, my partner, tried to be understanding, but at times I think he found it hard to comprehend the enormousness of what was going on in my head. I worried about being a good mum, the potential for postnatal depression, the pregnancy itself, and particularly labour and birth.

There was never any question in my mind about where we would have the baby. Home was where I wanted to be, especially after attending so many beautiful home births. However, mentally preparing for labour and birth was a big challenge for me, as it was something I always knew I would have to do but had always been afraid of. Being a midwife was a disadvantage, as I felt I knew too much and had to get my head around the 'what ifs'. I found it easier to focus on the birth once I had left work. The pressure to perform was lifted as I cocooned myself in the familiar environment of our beautiful home.

I finished work at 36 weeks, which was a great relief. By the end of it I found I was dragging myself around feeling absolutely exhausted. Nigel and I both felt that I would go into labour before my due date – 11 July – and I was thinking the baby would be born in June. I was getting Braxton Hicks contractions quite frequently and felt that the baby was very low, as I could feel it moving on my cervix. Any little pain I got, Nigel would say, 'Is this it?' excitedly wishing and hoping that it was. He also kept making me hot curries and massaging me with oils that are usually not recommended in pregnancy because they can bring on labour. We knew it would only work if I was ready, but it was fun anyway.

On 4 July I had a very busy day. Nigel was on holidays now and I had a list of cleaning to do, which I was meant to have done before his holiday so that we could enjoy our time together. Nigel was painting a mural in the nursery, so I took his girls, Erin (five) and Roisin (three), and did some shopping. When we got home I started on the cleaning and cleaned the kitchen from top to toe. I managed to get through everything except the vacuuming. By the end of it I had lower backache, which I passed off as being my usual lower back problem – nothing new. I was getting a lot of Braxton Hicks contractions and at around 10 pm I had some low period-type pain. I told Nigel and he teasingly said, 'If you're not in labour I don't want to know.' I said I didn't think I was and that I'd had a busy day. We went to bed at around 11 pm and I could feel the tightenings spacing out, so I thought, oh well, that's the end of that.

I had a restless night and was awake from 3 am to 6 am on and off. When I awoke at 7 am I lay there looking at the clock. The tightenings were still there but were not regular. Nigel got me breakfast in bed and I said I thought when I got up that they would probably get closer together – and they did. I got up at about 8 am and straightaway they kicked in. Nigel was keeping a close eye on me. He kept wanting to set everything up, but I said no in case it wasn't the real thing.

We had set up a tepee for the birth. Nigel kept himself busy starting the fire and setting up the mattress and bedding. At around 9 am I thought I should ring Natalie, the photographer, and give her early warning, and also Vicki, a midwife friend. Nigel needed to go to the shops to get some things. When he left I went into the tepee to keep an eye on the fire and spend some time on all fours to encourage the baby to be in an optimal position, as I still felt a lot of limbs at the front.

Nigel returned at around 10 am and by this time the tightenings were having some effect on me. They were fairly strong, but I was still able to walk through them. I went inside to finish my jobs, just in case this definitely was labour.

I went to the toilet and to my excitement I had a small show. I informed Nigel that yes, it was real, and he could finally set up the birth pool. So to the vacuuming I went. It was 11 am and I had just started in our bedroom when I got a strong tightening, which made me stop, and then I felt a warm gush. Knowing instantly what it was, I raced out of the room and called, 'Nigel!' at the top of my voice. It had given me such a fright and I thought I would have the baby really quickly. I was shaking as I sat on the toilet. I looked up at Nigel then down at the green liquor. My heart sank immediately. It was meconium and I was unsure if it was fresh or not. 'What will we do?' I asked Nigel. 'What do you want to do?' he asked me. I wanted to do what was best for the baby, but I could see our plans of a home birth going out the window, which was disappointing. I didn't want to make the decision. I wanted someone to tell me whether we should go to hospital or stay at home. I looked to Nigel for an answer and he said the right thing: 'I'm not your midwife. We'll have to ring Lynne.' We couldn't get hold of Lynne straightaway and left a message, so while I had a shower Nigel rang Vicki. He came back and said that Vicki felt it would be okay to stay at home for now. Nigel and I listened to the baby's heartbeat and it was beautiful and strong.

The contractions kicked in very quickly now and I found myself stopping and needing to concentrate. I was also humming loudly with each one. The girls had been playing in their room all this time, but while I was in the bathroom Roisin appeared at the door to see what was happening. 'The baby's coming today, Ro.' She disappeared. After the next contraction I looked up to see both her and Erin hovering near the doorway, giggling.

I went down to the tepee and lay on the mattress as the contractions relentlessly continued. I was enjoying this time and the realisation that this was really it. I was being very vocal and it felt good, although things seemed to be moving fast and I was anxious that Lynne, Vicki and Natalie wouldn't arrive on time.

Poor Nigel busied himself setting up the pool, stoking the fire, attending to the girls, answering the phone and making sure I was okay. I could see him ducking in and out of the tepee. Where was everyone? Natalie rang and I said to Nigel, 'Tell her to come now!' Photos and memories are very important to me, and I didn't want to miss anything.

I said to Nigel that I didn't think the pool would be ready in time because I could feel the baby just inside. I should have let him start preparing it earlier when he had wanted to.

Lynne arrived at 12.30 pm and I felt such relief. I'm sure Nigel did too. I told Lynne that I didn't think it would be long. Vicki and Natalie arrived soon afterwards. Yay, everyone was here!

The next few hours went by so quickly as the intensity of the labour took hold. It was not like I'd imagined it to be at all. I knew it would be painful, but I didn't know it would take over my whole body the way it did. We had bought some beautiful music, which I imagined I could lose myself in, but as loud as it was I didn't hear a word – I was in my own world.

The low abdominal pains were severe, but nothing like the excruciating back pain that enveloped me – it felt as though my back was breaking. The birth pool was a lost cause. Nigel struggled to get it filled, but the hot water was running out. Roisin amused herself with the water and Erin sat by my side with Vicki. I didn't know what to do. I couldn't keep still. I cried for hot towels, anything that would give me some relief. I wanted to be touched but when I was it was never the right place. Sometimes massage helped and at other times it was unbearable. Visualisation didn't work, as the intensity of labour was distracting and I couldn't let myself go anywhere else. A couple of times I felt like I would lose the plot, but somewhere I found strength to continue. Nigel was just wonderful, getting me drinks, massaging me, being there to hold onto and just loving me. He told me constantly that he loved me, but I couldn't always get the words out to say it back to him. I wanted to be close to him, but at the same time I felt smothered. It didn't help that the fire was raging so hard it felt as though it was 40°C. For a time, Nigel couldn't do a thing right. I remember looking up to see him coming in with more towels – a green one and one of my precious cream ones. 'Not the cream one!' I shouted. He then meekly put them on a chair and went to put some more wood on the fire. 'No more wood on the fire,' I cried. Poor Nigel!

I said to Lynne that I couldn't understand why it was taking so long. She reminded me about **caput** and **moulding**, to which I groaned. I lost all track of time as I was carried along the hard road to our baby. I again tried visualisation techniques, but found I couldn't keep the visions in my head as I needed to focus all my attention on getting through each contraction. I needed to concentrate on vocalisation, which I did with a vengeance. It felt fantastic to holler as loud as I could; I think it was my way of being in control. Before long, I had the vague urge to push and felt my body take control at the end of each contraction. Can I push? 'If you want to,' Lynne said. I didn't need encouragement. I just wanted it over now, so once I got the all clear, no one could stop me. Even though I wanted to push, I didn't like the sensation. Looking back, I think it was because I wasn't quite ready. It's hard to push when your body's not going with you.

After a time I needed a break, so Nigel and I went to the bathroom for a while. I sat on the toilet and it felt like a good position. Eventually we went back to the tepee. It was now 3.30 pm. Lynne said the baby was direct OP (posterior – looking face up), which was a surprise to me even though during the pregnancy this was the case. That would account for the excruciating back pain. The cervix was swollen but I was 8 centimetres dilated. Relief! Slightly disappointed that I wasn't fully dilated, I knew I had to try to stop the urge to push. Vicki suggested we do some hip swinging to try to encourage the baby to turn anterior. All I knew was that I would do anything if it helped me to stop pushing and speed things up. From somewhere I summoned up the strength to get to my feet. Boy, was that hard work! I hollered at the top of my voice like there was no tomorrow. It felt as though the louder I hollered the easier it was to get through each contraction. Eventually I tired and desperately wanted to use the bath. It was about 4 pm now.

The hot water was still an issue and the bath had to be filled by pans from the stove. It felt like an eternity before I was able to get in.

I eventually made it to the sanctuary of the bath, which was so hot that I nearly fainted. It was such a relief, though, and felt so soothing for my poor body. I found myself squatting as the urge to push became overbearing and my body just took over. All the while, Lynne was listening closely to the baby's heartbeat, as the meconium liquor had continued. At 4.30 pm Lynne suggested that she examine me again, just to check that I was fully dilated. I still had a swollen anterior lip of cervix left, which Lynne was able to push back easily with the next two contractions. The head came down past the cervix. At last it was definitely okay for me to push. I got up into a squat again and just pushed with all my might with each contraction. As much as I liked to be pushing, since I could feel the baby coming closer with each one, I still wanted to run away from it all. With each push I was convinced I was going to split in half. I was surprised at how quickly the head was coming.

At this point Nigel's aunt arrived to pick up the girls, as Nigel had phoned her. About 5 minutes later I felt the head coming and realised Nigel wasn't in the room. I called to him to come back, which he did, and after a couple more contractions our baby's head was born. It took me by surprise, as I remember consciously trying to let the head come out slowly to minimise trauma to my perineum, and I didn't think it would come out until the next contraction. I had my hand there the whole time and felt the baby's face as it came out. I reached down and felt cord around the baby's neck. I wanted Lynne to try to loop it over and she loosened it a little.

We waited for the next contraction and I felt as though I couldn't reach down far enough to catch the baby myself – I knew I wanted the baby to feel my or Nigel's touch first. Lynne put her hands down and I said, 'No, I want Nigel to birth the baby,' to which he initially said no. I felt a little panic. Well, who was going to catch this baby? I don't know what made Nigel change his mind, but he put his hands in the water. I had another contraction and with a final push our baby made a grand entrance into the world. Out of the water this huge bundle of joy came up to greet me face to face. I saw this purple/blue baby covered thickly in **vernix**, with large, shocked eyes staring at me. I couldn't believe it.

It was 5 pm – our baby was here at last and he was the most beautiful creature on earth. Even with his head very moulded from caput, and swelling off to the left side, he was beautiful, with the sweetest face. I couldn't get over his huge hands. I remember quickly pulling his legs apart to reveal that we had a little boy. Our prediction was right and I gasped with delight. 'It's Angus. It's an Angus.' I found myself crying with relief, exhaustion, happiness and overwhelming joy. I'd done it; I'd given birth! We lay down together in the bath to keep him warm and I tried to take it all in. No more back pain – I was ecstatic. Within twenty minutes, Angus was suckling happily at my breast. He was a natural.

After a while I went to the toilet and at 6.15 pm I birthed the placenta. While we were waiting, Nigel sat on the floor with Angus and we relived the day's events. We went back to the tepee for celebrations. It was dark now and the tepee was lovely and warm. I lay on the mattress and Nigel, Lynne, Vicki and I toasted each other and Angus with champagne and chocolates. Welcome to the world!

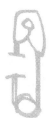

Early versus late cord clamping

Early clamping of the baby's umbilical cord can mean your newborn infant does not receive that extra placental blood that could help him or her in the first few minutes of life. Before your baby was born, blood flowed freely between the baby and its placenta. If the umbilical cord is clamped before it has stopped pulsating, the baby doesn't receive that blood still in the cord and placenta. Many women now prefer to wait until the cord has stopped pulsating before having it cut.

If a woman is given Syntocinon to speed up the delivery of the placenta, the baby will usually have to have its cord cut and clamped immediately. In most cases, however, a woman's body will produce hormones and contractions to expel the placenta. The baby suckling at the woman's breast will also speed up this process, and in most cases there is no need to use Syntocinon to hasten delivery of the placenta.

If the cord is not clamped until it has stopped pulsating, the baby receives valuable extra blood – up to 40 per cent of the baby's blood volume. The baby also continues to receive oxygen from the cord and is not forced to take oxygen into his or her lungs immediately. This can be less traumatic for your baby.

Another benefit to a baby is the bonding and lack of separation from the mother possible in the time immediately following birth. Babies tend to have lower haemoglobin levels when early cord clamping is initiated.

Natural **third stage** (delivery of the placenta) is carried out by some midwives in birth centres and at home births, and sometimes at the request of the mother.

Early versus late cord clamping is continually scrutinised, and you need to discuss the pros and cons with your birth professional. Individual assessment of each person makes for the best decision.

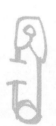

Vaginal birth after caesarean

Vaginal birth after caesarean, or VBAC as it is commonly known, is becoming more frequent. Less than a decade ago it was not encouraged, and it was considered that once a woman had had a caesarean then all subsequent births had to be surgical births. Thanks to improvements in surgical techniques, the discontinuation of poor birth practices and the work of dedicated midwives, more and more women are choosing a vaginal birth for their next child.

One of the major fears with a vaginal birth following a caesarean is a ruptured uterus. This was more of a problem when the incision for the caesarean was made vertically. In most cases today, the incision is smaller, lower and horizontal (transverse). This has allowed VBAC with greater safety.

For those women who felt dismayed and disappointed after the caesarean birth of their child, VBAC is now an option, depending on the reason for the previous caesarean. You need to find out as much as you can about VBAC and be prepared to commit yourself to it. Finding a doctor or midwife prepared to support your aspirations is important, and planning ahead with them will aid in making you feel relaxed and comfortable about your decision. A healthy diet and a suitable exercise program will help to increase your chances of a trouble-free birth.

Having experienced a problem once, some women feel safer choosing a caesarean for their next birth, and this is right for them. However, it is wonderful to know that there is now a real choice for those who wish to have a normal birth.

Dianne's third birth story

Yes, that was definitely another contraction I just felt. It was midday on a Saturday and I was at home with my husband, Brett, and our two children, Sophie and Lucy. Today was the day my baby was due.

Deciding to do nothing, I ignored the contraction as best I could. As I was 38 and it was my third child, I had some expectations as to how my labour might go. This time around, I definitely had a plan. My two previous births had both been very high-tech, big-city hospital deliveries by caesarean, surrounded by obstetricians and anaesthetists. This time I was determined it would be different. Having moved to a small country town, I was looking forward to giving birth in a small hospital with the local GP of my choice, and I was determined not to go to the hospital too soon.

The reason for my strong feelings was that with each of my two previous deliveries I had been in hospital two days prior to each birth, both of which had entailed more than two-day labours. Consequently, I was planning to leave for hospital at the last possible moment.

My pains continued all day, but I relaxed as best I could. By 8.30 pm, four-and-a-half-year-old Sophie was kissing me good night, and I said, 'Ouch!'

'What is the matter, Mummy?' Sophie asked, and I told her our baby was letting me know it would soon be ready to be born. I then took two sleeping tablets (prearranged by my doctor) and went straight to bed (in the hope of ignoring these overnight niggly pains).

An hour and a half later, I was woken up by strong, crampy pains. The next five hours were spent sitting at the dining table, surrounded by a quilt and lots of pillows, trying to be as upright as possible, but also able to rest. By 3.30 am, Brett came out from our bedroom. 'Come back to bed, darling,' he said, but I couldn't and so he stayed up rubbing my back, talking to me and trying his best to help.

At about 6 am, Brett and I decided to wake up our children to take them to a friend's place. Our plan was to nip into the hospital to check on my progress, and then come home again. We just wanted to see if my all-night contractions had opened my cervix at all. So, at 7.30 am on a very frosty morning, we set off for the hospital, thinking what it would be like to have a chilly winter's baby. At the hospital I was examined and to my amazement I was found to be 4 to 5 centimetres dilated. I was thrilled. I was told I could go home if I wanted to, but it wasn't too early to stay. Hearing this, we decided to stay.

At 8.30 am, I was looked at by a doctor. Everything was fine. Then, at 9.30 am, Brett decided he wanted to time my contractions, just to see how far apart they were. I wasn't interested. I refused to acknowledge any details just yet, as I felt the baby still had a long time in coming. By 10 am I was given another examination, which found me to be 7 centimetres dilated. I was told I was doing well. Starting to become excited, I thought to myself, no, no, no – don't get too excited, it's still early days yet.

The next few hours I spent wandering up and down the corridor. By 2.30 pm I was 9.5 centimetres dilated, but an examination at 3.15 pm showed our baby's head was still high, with a little rim of cervix yet to open. It was then that I decided I needed pain relief and was given a mask of **nitrous oxide** from which I could breathe. This was the first pain relief I had taken so far, but I couldn't get it to work properly. I had to breathe in the gas so deeply to feel it coming out that I would go dizzy between contractions, so I stopped taking it.

Another examination at 4 pm showed I still had half a centimetre of cervix yet to open. The doctor decided that, if I hadn't had the baby by the time it got dark, he would insert a Syntocinon drip to speed things up.

All day long I had been having trouble going to the toilet. Nevertheless, at 5.15 pm, I had this comical impression come to my mind. Our baby was sending me a message: 'Have one last try at the toilet, Mum.' So I did. While squirming around on the toilet seat, this last lip of cervix finally opened. The baby saw his chance, headed straight for the opening and I felt his head just drop. I let out a blood-curdling shriek, which the nurse immediately recognised as a sign of imminent delivery. She called the doctor, but unfortunately the phone was engaged and it took her several minutes to get through. In the meantime, another midwife appeared out of nowhere as I slowly struggled back to my bed.

Now fully dilated, I started pushing. It was a wonderful feeling. Then, just as the midwife was about to start delivering, in flew the doctor, who promptly took over. 'Push, push,' came the doctor's voice, as everyone crowded around to watch the head emerge. Then, with one final push, out slithered our beautiful son.

Michael was born at 5.30 pm. He weighed 3660 grams and was 50.2 centimetres long. Soon after he was born, I had a shower, which I just couldn't believe. With my two previous births, I had been recovering from an epidural anaesthetic immediately following delivery, and couldn't move, or get out of bed, until well into the next day.

I walked or floated back to my room. Here I was having just given birth to my son – and naturally. No caesarean and no epidural. I finally felt I had really given birth. It didn't even worry me that I had had a couple of stitches (because of Michael turning his head sideways as he was being born).

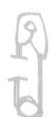

Getting ready for your baby

You will likely enjoy getting ready for the birth of your baby – putting things together into drawers, then taking from your 'baby things' for your pre-packed hospital bag. An important thing to remember is that this is an individual matter. For example, some people will want four button-down-the-front nighties for breastfeeding and one baby singlet for every day of the week. Others will make do with two nighties and four singlets as they wash so frequently they only need that number. This having been said, here is a suggested list of what you will need. Increase the baby items accordingly if you are having a multiple birth.

- 7 stretch suits size 000
- 7 stretch suits size 00
- 7 singlets size 00
- 5 small baby blankets for wrapping up baby
- 4 large cot blankets for baby's cot
- 5 packets newborn-size disposable nappies, or 2 or 3 dozen cloth nappies and nappy pins
- 4 pairs of socks or booties
- 1 jar of Vaseline to help avoid nappy rash
- 1 jar/tube of sorbelene or glycerine cream to soothe dry, irritated skin
- 7 plastic-backed bibs
- 1 bottle of baby-bath solution (newborn age)
- 1 bottle of baby shampoo
- 1 tube/bottle of baby lotion
- 1 pack of cotton buds
- 4 soft towels
- 10 face washers to bath baby and wipe baby's bottom at nappy-change time
- 40 terry towelling bibs to pick up spills from vomiting babies. These can also be used as baby wipes at nappy-change time, and can be bleached before washing for extra hygiene
- 1 shoulder carrybag for going out with baby
- 1 change mat
- disposable bags to hold dirty nappies to keep in your carry bag

Labour kit

Out of the above, you can put in your hospital bag:

- 1 size 000 baby stretch suit
- 1 size 00 singlet

- ◊ 1 pair of baby socks or booties
- ◊ 1 small baby blanket to wrap the baby to come home in (the hospital will provide nappies for your baby during your stay, and also sanitary napkins)
- ◊ 1 baby capsule, fitted into your car
- ◊ 3 nursing nighties for you
- ◊ 3 nursing bras
- ◊ 1 pair of comfortable day clothes suitable for breastfeeding
- ◊ 5 pairs clean underwear
- ◊ 1 packet sanitary napkins
- ◊ 1 packet nursing pads
- ◊ 1 pair of slippers or comfortable shoes
- ◊ 1 pair of clothes for going home in
- ◊ pencil and paper
- ◊ list of phone numbers
- ◊ change for the telephone, chocolate, snacks, etc.
- ◊ toiletries, toothbrush, soap, face washer, etc.
- ◊ box of tissues
- ◊ empty bag for rubbish
- ◊ optional: cards to announce the arrival of your baby (stamps, envelopes, etc.)

Depending on where you are giving birth and the arrangements you have made with your support people, you may have additional items that you will be taking with you, such as music, cameras, massage oils and so on.

part three

Birth process and labour

By the end of their pregnancy, most women begin to get excited at the prospect of finally meeting their baby. For some, this is an unknown experience, but even for experienced mums you can never be quite sure how it will go. The following stories and information should prepare you for this exciting time in your life, and help you to avoid some of the more painful and difficult experiences of labour.

Ways to identify the start of labour

As the birth approaches, a woman's body begins to prepare for the labour. Signs that women may experience prior to labour include:

- show (pink mucous discharge from the vagina), indicating engagement of the baby's head
- more frequent Braxton Hicks contractions
- a change in baby's movements as he or she runs out of space
- weight loss of up to 1 kilogram
- low pelvic pressure due to baby's position
- some diarrhoea
- nesting behaviour (some women experience a surge in energy just prior to the birth).

Once the conditions are right, labour will commence. Science still has not identified the actual triggers that cause labour to start. Once labour has started, the hormone **oxytocin** is responsible for causing the uterus to have strong, regular contractions. A centre in the woman's brain triggers the release of oxytocin. Real labour contractions feel very different from the Braxton Hicks contractions that women experience during pregnancy. The most important difference is that labour contractions come regularly, while Braxton Hicks contractions come irregularly. A contraction during labour starts gradually, builds to a peak, then fades away. Typically, when labour begins, the contractions are short in length, around 20 to 30 seconds. As labour progresses, contractions become gradually longer and stronger. Contractions need to be approximately 60 seconds long to really start to dilate or open the cervix. Labour contractions can last up to 90 seconds. When a woman gets true labour contractions they take all of her concentration and she is unable to talk through them.

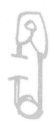

Stages of labour

L abour has three stages, simply known as the first, second and third stages of labour. During the first stage, the mouth of the uterus, called the cervix, goes from being closed to fully open (dilated to 10 centimetres). Strong, regular contractions of the uterus cause the cervix to open.

During the second stage of labour, the baby moves down the birth canal and is born. Women in this stage of labour assist the birth of the baby by pushing during the contractions. The third stage of labour begins after the baby is born and ends with the birth of the placenta and membranes (afterbirth).

The first stage of labour usually starts slowly, with mild cramping or a continuous ache. This may fade out or continue to grow, with the contractions gaining in strength and frequency. They may come every twenty to 30 minutes or be more erratic. You will know that true labour has begun when the contractions are coming every five to ten minutes and are growing in length and intensity. The cervix will have begun to thin (efface) and dilate. Once the contractions are coming every three to five minutes they will also have grown in strength and be lasting up to one minute. Hopefully you are now several centimetres dilated. This is now the time to leave for the hospital or birth centre if you have not already done so. The time you plan to leave depends on you and the distance to your hospital. Going too early means a long wait at the hospital and the chance that the labour may stop and you must come home again. If you know that you have quick births, if it is your first time or you feel uncertain, go earlier. Feeling safe and relaxed is better for your labour.

All labours are different and the dilation of the cervix can be quick in the beginning, reaching 6 or 7 centimetres in a matter of hours only to take a long time to fully dilate. Some are slow but regular while others are slow to reach the midway point, then pleasantly surprise the mother by being fast to reach complete dilation.

The contractions will eventually be coming every one to two minutes and may last for a minute. There should be a respite of a minute or two before the next contraction, but not always. The final part of the first stage is called transition. The contractions at this time are extremely intense as the cervix finally fully dilates and the baby's head begins to enter the birth canal.

The second stage of labour is the descent of the baby down the birth canal. This is when you are finally able to start pushing with each contraction. Many women feel a great relief to be able to push at this time. The second stage usually takes one to two hours, though it can take as little as five minutes. As the baby's head comes down the canal, the mother's coccyx moves to allow the head to pass through. Once the head moves fully into the birth canal, it can be seen and felt at the vaginal opening. You may feel a burning sensation as the perineum stretches to allow the head to pass through. Stopping at this stage to give the perineum time to stretch completely will help you avoid a tear or the need for an episiotomy. Your birth attendant may gently place his or her hand against the baby's head to prevent it coming through, and the panting you may have been practising in birth classes should now be done.

Now it is time to push your baby out. First the head will emerge, followed by the shoulders and the rest of the body. The contractions will stop almost immediately and you will hopefully have your baby placed directly onto your stomach. The cord is then cut and the baby taken to have its Apgar scores, weight and measurement recorded.

The third stage is the delivery of the placenta. This can take an hour but usually no longer. Syntocinon may be given to speed up the process, but unless there are medical reasons, there is no reason not to let nature take its course.

Jocelyn's birth story

This was my first baby. I was nineteen when I fell pregnant, but had turned twenty by the time I was nine months pregnant.

At 1.35 am I began to feel pains, but I wasn't sure what was happening so I went to the toilet, where I lost a bit of pinkish-coloured blood. I got Mum out of bed and told her what was happening.

'It's hurting every five minutes and there was some blood when I went to the toilet,' I confided. 'You're in labour,' she explained, 'but it will be a while yet. Just wait.'

By 3.30 am, the pains were coming every three and a half minutes. I decided to go to the hospital. The ten-minute trip was very exciting. My contractions were coming regularly but were not too painful. I was nervous, but also very happy, thinking, 'If this is all there is to labour, I can easily handle it'. (Little did I realise!)

When we arrived at the hospital I was given a white hospital gown to put on. I was examined and found to be more than halfway dilated (about 6 centimetres). My waters were broken during the examination (they had already leaked a little). Then the pain really started.

To cope with the very strong pains, I decided to have a hot shower. The water was so comforting I could hardly feel the pains any more. Consequently, I stayed in there for the next one and a half hours, until a midwife came and asked me to get out. Reluctantly I left the shower and the contractions once again became almost unbearable. With the midwife's help, I managed to walk from the shower back to the examination room. It was 5.30 am. Here I was examined and found to be fully dilated. Next, several staff lifted me off my bed and onto a bed with wheels, so I could be pushed into the delivery ward. The midwife then asked if I felt like pushing. 'I think so,' I replied, 'but I'm not too sure.'

For the next hour and twenty minutes I pushed with every contraction that came. They were coming every two minutes and were extremely painful. I tried some gas but it didn't work, apart from on one occasion where all it did was make me feel faint and weaker than I was.

Everyone present began encouraging me as best they could. 'You're almost there ... Come on, push ... push,' came the midwife's voice.

'I can see the head,' came my partner's voice.

'Look, look, the hair is black,' my little sister's excited voice cried out.

'Of course the hair would be black,' I thought. (Try and I are of Asian descent.)

Finally, the doctor decided she had to give me an episiotomy and asked if she could do this. I was very reluctant, but once the cut was done it made a big difference and I was finally able to push our baby out. The head came out, soon followed by the rest of the baby's body.

Our baby boy was born at 7.01 am, weighing 3020 grams, and was 50.5 centimetres long. His Apgar scores at birth were 9 and then 10. The pain was now over and we now had our gorgeous baby son, Rocky.

Carol's third birth story

'How big do you think this baby will be?' I asked, anxiously anticipating the doctor's reply. 'Yes, this baby is going to be smaller than your first two. It will be about 2500 grams.'

Four days later, ten days before my due date (of Christmas Day), I had a heavy cold. Regardless of this, I decided to take up my teenaged niece's offer to babysit our two little girls while I went out for the evening.

'I think you are definitely having this baby soon,' said my sister Patricia as she looked intently into my eyes. 'Your eyes have that glazed-over faraway look they always get when you are about to deliver a baby.'

'Really?' I said, not completely agreeing with her, but hoping that she might be correct.

Later that evening at home, I began to believe my sister could be right. I couldn't sleep, so several hours later jumped out of bed when I felt my first contraction. It was 3.45 am. My two previous births had been very fast: Amanda three and a half hours, and Samantha one hour and ten minutes, so I felt a sense of urgency.

Quickly I put my birth plan into action. I rang my friend and sister-in-law, Mary, and told her to meet us at the hospital. Next I went and woke up Clem, who promptly rolled over and went back to sleep. So much for a nervous, panicky husband! It took me a further twenty minutes and a cup of coffee to coax him out of bed.

Now fully awake, Clem ran next door to wake up his mum, who was to look after our children. While he did this, I rushed around collecting last-minute things to take in my already-packed hospital bag. When my mother-in-law arrived, Clem drove me straight to the hospital.

Even the routine procedure of filling out forms at the hospital desk didn't take away the excitement of knowing I would soon be holding this baby in my arms. Mary joined us after my initial examination. The three of us went into the first-stage room [not available in all hospitals], comfortably equipped with lounge chairs, a television, bathroom and kitchen. The atmosphere was just right for an enjoyable chat – apart from my regular, painful one-minute contractions coming every few minutes.

For the next two hours, Mary and Clem took turns comforting me through every pain. By 6.30 am I called out to a passing midwife to examine me, but was disappointed when I was found to be only 3 centimetres dilated. I asked if she could break my waters to speed things up, but she refused, saying this could in fact slow things down.

One hour later, I once again asked the midwife to rupture my membranes, explaining how my two previous labours had only progressed once my waters had been broken. By now I had been in labour for nearly four hours. The nurse gave in and took me to the examination room where she brought out an instrument looking very much like a crochet hook with a long handle. With this she broke my waters. I was still only 3 centimetres dilated.

Within minutes of having my membranes ruptured, I sensed I was dilating quickly and asked to be moved to the delivery suite. Fifty minutes and about fifteen contractions later, I was fully dilated.

A few minutes later, at 8.25 am, after several long pushes, I gave birth to our third beautiful daughter, Mary Elizabeth. She weighed 3470 grams and was 52 centimetres long. When handed our baby for the first time, my thought was, 'She's beautiful'. I also felt a sense of pride and disbelief that Clem and I now had three children, and all in less than three years.

I needn't have worried about the doctor telling me how small our baby was going to be, because she was our biggest yet – and only days after that examination. I also need not have worried about having a short labour, as this turned out to be my longest, lasting four hours and 40 minutes, although I do believe it would have been shorter had my waters been broken earlier.

Length of labour

The length of labour is very difficult to anticipate. The average length for first-time mothers is around twelve to fourteen hours for the first stage of labour and one to two hours for the second stage of labour. Generally, women expecting their second or subsequent baby can anticipate a shorter labour than their first. However, it is important to keep an open mind, as anything is possible. Labour may exceed the average, and as long as mother and baby are fine there is no problem with this. The length of labour depends on many different factors, including the baby's position (some positions are better than others at stimulating contractions) and the size and strength of the contractions. The midwife or doctor will monitor the progress of the labour and may recommend strategies to help manage a long labour.

Donna's second birth story – a fast birth

Donna had had a short stay in hospital for blood pressure but had been allowed home. Her story continues from Part 1.

It was the third of September and I was due to have the baby on the seventeenth. At 10.30 pm I started getting a sharp pain as I was walking up the stairs. 'Uh-oh,' I said to my uncle, who was visiting us at the time. 'This could be it.'

Half an hour later the pains were coming every five minutes, so I rang the hospital and was asked, 'Do you think you should come in?'

'Yes, I think I'd better,' I replied.

Then, while I was still talking on the phone, my pains started coming every two minutes. So here I was waiting for my husband, Steve, to get home, but he didn't arrive. Instead, my uncle ended up taking me to the hospital. Luke, my little boy, was also with us.

When I got to the hospital, the midwife discovered that I was 8 centimetres dilated. 'You're going to have this baby any moment,' she told me.

Not long after we arrived, Steve joined me. The labour itself was very painful, with my contractions coming every two minutes and with only a minute's break between them. It was progressing so quickly that I didn't have time for pain relief (which was good).

As with my first labour, my waters didn't break by themselves and had to be broken. This was done just before I was told to start pushing.

After one hour in hospital, I was fully dilated. With my next contraction, I was told to start pushing and was told they could see the head coming.

My body didn't want to cooperate, as everything was happening so quickly. My baby was in a hurry to be born and was coming faster than I could comfortably cope with. The next thing I knew, the midwife said to me, 'Your baby's head is out, just relax.' And that's when she said, 'You can pull your baby out now.'

'Oh no,' I thought, saying, 'What if I accidentally hurt him?' But she said, 'No, you'll manage.' So I put my hands under his little arms and simply lifted him out. As I pulled my baby out, he was facing me, so straight away I said, 'It's a boy!' It was so amazing and so easy, and all I could think was, 'Wow.'

Our baby was placed on my stomach until the cord had stopped pulsating. Steve was asked if he wanted to cut it but he was concerned he might hurt the baby, and was very worried when a small amount of blood came out. Our baby was fine and I was able pick him up and feed him.

Birthing your own baby

Many women will reach down with their hand and touch their baby's head as it first emerges. It is also possible for a woman who has almost finished delivering to birth her own baby. As the baby's body emerges, a woman may be able to reach down, grasp the baby under the armpits and bring it up into her arms.

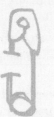

Long labour

For first-time mothers the average labour lasts about thirteen to sixteen hours. Subsequent deliveries take about eight hours. Sometimes, however, labour may progress very slowly or even come to a standstill. Some reasons for a long labour include:

- the mother's contractions are not effective
- the baby is in a posterior position (the back of the baby's head is against the woman's spine, instead of its face towards it)
- the baby's head is very large and does not easily fit into its mother's pelvis
- the baby is lying in a face, breech or brow presentation.

In the case of a long labour, a Syntocinon drip can be started to speed contractions and, in some cases, the woman's membranes will need to be ruptured first. Epidurals are frequently offered to a woman experiencing a long labour, enabling her to rest. This also means she is prepared should she need an emergency caesarean.

Dianne's second birth story

Having reached full term, I was at home with my husband, Brett, and our two-year-old daughter, Sophie. It was 3 pm when I experienced what felt like a cramp. Wanting to be by myself, I lay down and eventually fell asleep.

Awoken by another cramp, I thought, 'Here goes – this must be the beginning of my labour.' I decided to go for a walk around the block to relieve the crampy contractions. These contractions continued at home, but by 6 pm I became confused because they were coming so frequently yet were so mild. I rang the hospital and was told to wait for an hour and then to ring back.

At 8.30 pm I rang back, and was told they had contacted my doctor because of my previous caesarean. My doctor thought that I should go straight to the hospital to see what was happening. Brett drove me to the hospital after first putting Sophie to bed where friends would look after her.

Upon arrival at the hospital, I had to answer some questions and was then taken to the labour ward, where I had to change into a white hospital gown. The midwife then hooked me up to a fetal monitoring machine and gave me an examination. It was now 9.45 pm. I was found to be 1 centimetre dilated and the midwives told me that they didn't think anything much was going to happen.

'I think I might just go home then,' I replied. 'Oh, no,' came the reply. 'Your doctor said you should stay.'

Brett then came with me to the first-stage room, where we ended up staying until 11.30 pm. At that time, a nurse came to tell me that there were plenty of empty beds in the delivery ward. Did I want to go there and lie down, as I might get some better rest? Thinking this sounded like a good idea, I went. The contractions were now becoming more irregular. They were still mild, but strong enough to prevent me from sleeping. I stayed in the delivery ward all night, dozing between contractions, but by morning felt as though I hadn't slept at all.

At 9.20 am a doctor came to examine me. After all-night contractions coming every five to ten minutes, I was still only 1 centimetre dilated. The doctor told me he would induce me the following morning if nothing more had happened, but I was still not allowed to go home. He then suggested I go back to the labour ward. In the meantime, Brett had gone to work after having been in the hospital all night.

My contractions were now all over the place – every twenty minutes, then eight minutes, then three minutes apart – just frequent enough that I could never really rest. So I spent the whole day pacing the corridors of the maternity ward. By 9 pm I thought I would look into the nursery and get some inspiration. But instead I became upset and began to cry. At about the same time, my waters broke and my pains became slightly stronger and more frequent. Things were finally going to happen (or so I thought).

By 11.30 pm I was asked if I wanted some sleeping tablets. I had by now been away from home for 24 hours without proper sleep, and I knew I would definitely be having this baby tomorrow, naturally or not.

So I said yes, but one hour after I finally fell asleep I was awoken because the pains were becoming so strong. Forty-five minutes later, a sister from the labour ward was sent to examine me and I was found to be 3 centimetres dilated. I had been in labour for almost one and a half days, and this was all I had to show for it.

The contractions were now so painful that, after speaking to the sister, I went to the labour ward to get a mask of nitrous oxide. I stayed on the gas until 6 am, breathing it in when I needed to relieve the pain. At the same time, my baby was being monitored.

At about 7 am Brett arrived, then at 8.15 am the doctor came in. After finding me 4 centimetres dilated, the doctor told the nurse to set up the drip. I asked the doctor if I could have an epidural, to which he agreed. The nurse then attempted to start my drip. The needle was pierced into my arm but missed my vein, so she pulled it out and tried again. Once again the needle didn't go in properly and once again she pulled it out. One last try – it missed my vein. So the nurse withdrew the needle and promptly walked off the job.

At 11 am, my induction and epidural still hadn't been set up and I was experiencing very painful contractions. As well as this, all the waiting, contractions and lack of sleep had begun to take their toll, and I was beginning to feel very distressed. The midwife realised this and decided to check on our baby, putting an internal electrode onto its head. Fortunately our baby was found to be fine, but the electrode was left in place so our baby could be continually monitored.

At 11.20 am the anaesthetist came to insert my epidural. When he saw that the drip was not inserted, he commented on this and then put it straight in without any problems whatsoever. But then the trouble started. While trying to insert the epidural, the anaesthetist hit a bone in my back, so had to stop and withdraw the tube. The second time too much blood came into the tube and this attempt had to be aborted. By the third stab into my back, the epidural was correctly positioned and the medication inserted. What a relief it was.

A solution of saline and glucose was then put into my drip and my blood pressure was checked to see how the epidural was affecting it. By 12.30 pm, the induction itself was finally started – Syntocinon was put into my drip. This hopefully meant that my labour would be sped up. Because of the epidural, I was now able to sleep, as I couldn't feel the pain from my contractions, but was awoken at 2 pm for an examination. I was found to be 6.5 centimetres dilated. Hooray, something was finally happening, I thought.

Half an hour later I realised I hadn't been to the toilet since 6 am but, because of the epidural, I couldn't feel which muscles to push, so a catheter had to be inserted. Five minutes later I was given a top-up of the epidural, which was still giving me great relief and enabling me to sleep.

At 3.45 pm the baby's trace fell off and a midwife had to put it back on. I was discovered to be 8.5 centimetres dilated. Then, only 35 minutes later, at 4.20 pm, I was found to be fully dilated. The doctor now told me I could begin to push, but then promptly left the room. Fortunately, Brett was still with me. He had been supporting me since 7 am, having only nipped out at lunchtime to get a bite to eat.

I was just about to start pushing when I remembered you have to push with a contraction, so I had Brett have a look at the monitor to let me know when I was having one. I couldn't feel them because I was numb from my waist down. With each contraction the nurse told me to push (which I was able to do four times into every one).

For the next twenty minutes I attempted to push our baby out, until the doctor came back to look at what was happening. He informed us that the baby's head was stuck, and twisted sideways.

I became very frightened for our baby. The doctor then said he would have to turn the baby's head with a pair of Keillands rotations forceps and, because of the size of these particular forceps, a larger-than-usual episiotomy would have to be done.

After witnessing this procedure, Brett left the room. He had seen enough already, and taking one look at that horrible instrument had to leave. It looked like some gruesome kind of tennis racket, with a very long handle. After the doctor finished, Brett came back in.

'Well, I'll just give you one last chance to push your baby out,' the doctor said. 'If you can't manage, I'll have to use the forceps.' I began to push with all my might.

Because I was numb and pushing so hard, I could feel the pressure in my head. After seven long pushes into the same contraction, I felt as though my head was coming off. But it must have been working, because finally our baby's head came out, followed quickly by its body (and without the help of forceps).

Our baby was placed straight onto my stomach and I heard someone say, 'It's a girl. And a good size, too.'

Lucy weighed 3850 grams and was 54 centimetres long. She was born at 4.50 pm, after more than two days of labour. Although my labour had actually lasted for more than 48 hours, the hospital only counted it as being a sixteen-hour labour. It took me 27 hours to dilate from 1 centimetre to 3 centimetres and then sixteen hours to dilate from 3 centimetres until birth.

Somehow, through all the drama, our darling Lucy had managed not to become distressed, and I will never forget that amazing feeling of skin-to-skin contact as my warm little newborn nestled on my tummy and looked into my eyes.

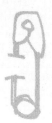

Electronic fetal monitoring

Electronic fetal monitoring is used to continuously record the baby's heartbeat. This may be done externally with two large elastic belts that are placed over the woman's abdomen: one belt holds the transducer that listens to the baby's heartbeat, and the other holds the tocodynamometer, which records uterine contractions. These readings are then recorded onto a piece of paper. Monitoring may also be carried out internally by attaching an electrode to the baby's scalp. This can only be done if the cervix is open a little and the membranes have been broken.

Electronic fetal monitoring may be used if the baby is showing signs of distress, during medical procedures (such as an epidural block or induction of labour), and if there are concerns for the baby's wellbeing, for example if the baby is premature or has a medical condition. Research has shown that electronic fetal monitoring has no benefit in a normal labour.

Problems with electronic fetal monitoring include immobilising the woman, difficulty interpreting the printout from the machine by health-care professionals, the machine rather than the woman becoming the focus of care, and increased chance of caesarean or forceps birth. If **internal monitoring** is used, there is an increased risk of the baby experiencing an infection or even having a laceration where the electrode was attached to the baby's scalp.

Waters breaking

In about 10 to 15 per cent of labours the waters will break before any contractions have occurred. For most women, however, the waters will break towards the end of the first stage or in the second stage of labour. When the waters break they should be clear. If they are stained green or brown in colour it could be that the baby has had a bowel motion in the waters. The first thing a woman should do if her waters break is to put on a sanitary pad to check the colour of the fluid. It is important then to contact a health-care professional. In about 90 per cent of cases when the waters break before labour begins, a woman will go into labour within 48 hours. Sometimes the waters do not break and the midwife or health-care practitioner may break them, although this is not always necessary. In cases where the waters break and labour does not follow within 48 hours, the baby may have to be induced to prevent the possibility of an infection reaching the baby.

Liz's birth story

Irritated, feeling enormous and simply tired of being pregnant, I found the doctor's words very comforting. 'You won't have to go on much longer,' he said, looking at my enormous stomach. It didn't help that I was past 40 weeks and had gained 16 kilograms.

In fact, my doctor proved to be wrong. Two and a half weeks later, still pregnant, I went to bed as usual, but awoke at 1 am feeling very thirsty. After having a drink, I went to the toilet, then back to bed, but by 2 am still hadn't managed to get back to sleep. Then my waters just erupted. Our double bed was absolutely flooded. Waking up my husband, Steve, I told him what had happened.

'Are you sure?' Steve replied, half asleep, as I lay in a pool of water.

'Feel it.' I said, putting Steve's hand into the wetness.

Now he awoke in an awful hurry, got out of bed and went straight to the phone to ring the hospital.

'My wife's waters have broken.' he told the midwife.

'Don't worry,' she replied. 'Your wife has a long way to go yet.'

Steve was so nervous, though, that we decided to go to the hospital right away. By now I was beginning to experience back pain. Upon arrival at the hospital I was examined and found to be 8 centimetres dilated. My baby was coming very quickly. My back contractions were still coming every five minutes. I didn't have to be flat on my back with my feet up in stirrups, as I had done nine years earlier with my first baby. I preferred being on my side while my baby was monitored.

I overheard the midwives saying that the baby's heartbeat was 152, and that it was probably a girl.* I was annoyed to hear them say this, as I wanted the sex of our baby to be a surprise.

The pain was now terrible. I requested drugs to relieve it, but was refused them because everything was progressing too quickly. Now in a world of my own, I was concentrating on handling the pain. I could hear other women screaming from other wards and was very disturbed by this. Not long after, my doctor was called to examine me. He looked as though he had just woken up. His shirt was crumpled and his hair was all ruffled. 'You are going to have to push,' he told me after finding me fully dilated. 'Your baby is in distress.'

The doctor also thought I might be having a big baby so decided to give me a hand. He got on one side of me, then had Steve go to the other, and I now had to push against the two of them, as hard as I could. It was very tiring and took me more than twenty minutes (about eight contractions) to deliver our baby's head. The pushing seemed to go on forever and was the hardest part of my labour.

Finally, the baby's head was out. It was 5.30 am, only three and half hours since my waters had broken. One shoulder followed, but then the baby became stuck. The doctor had to yank the baby by its stuck shoulder until it emerged. The rest of the baby then followed quickly.

'It's a girl – and big!' the doctor and midwife both said.

---

* Recent research indicates that there is no difference between the heart rate of boy and girl babies.

Our baby was taken away to have her nose and chest cleared. She was also weighed, measured and cleaned up before being brought back to us. 'She's 4150 grams, and 53 centimetres long,' we were told.

Jade was put onto my stomach and felt like a sack of potatoes. After a few minutes she was taken off again, wrapped up, then given to her proud daddy, Steve, who was overjoyed!

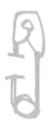

Artificial rupture of the membranes

Artificial rupture of the membranes is a procedure whereby the midwife or doctor artificially breaks the sac of amniotic fluid surrounding the baby using an instrument similar in appearance to a crochet hook. If this procedure is performed once the cervix is 3 (or more) centimetres dilated, it should not be painful. You will feel a gush of warm liquid. However, contractions will become more intense once the membranes have ruptured. The main reasons for performing artificial rupture of the membranes are to speed up labour, as a method of bringing on labour, and to see what colour the amniotic fluid is. The colour of the amniotic fluid should be clear or slightly pink. Sometimes the fluid is green or brown, indicating that the baby may have passed meconium. This is known as meconium staining. If the amniotic fluid is stained with thick meconium, there is greater cause for concern than if the fluid is only lightly stained. Meconium can indicate that the baby is in distress, but many babies pass meconium in the uterus simply because they are physcially able to do so.

If labour has started naturally, research has found that artificially rupturing the membranes can shorten labour by an average of one hour, but it can make contractions more painful and may increase the need for pain relief. Once the membranes have been ruptured, there is an increased risk of infection for the baby. Time limits may then be placed on the labour. If the labour is slow to progress, it may be accelerated by the introduction of hormones.

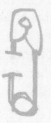

Labouring positions

Positions during labour can make a huge difference to the amount of pain a woman experiences. For example, if you are on your back, you actually reduce the efficiency of your contractions and increase the pain you may experience. Professor Mendez-Bauer discovered that dilation of the cervix and the efficiency of contractions is much greater when a woman is standing than when she is on her back, and that a woman experiences less pain if she is upright. A woman labouring flat on her back is lying on her **sacrum**, preventing the birth canal from opening as efficiently as it would if she were standing. A smaller opening also means more likelihood of problems while the child is being born, making it more likely that the woman will need medical intervention, such as an episiotomy. There are many positions you can adopt which will enable you to remain upright – squatting, sitting on a birth stool or toilet seat, walking around or leaning forward against an object such as the back of a chair.

Carol's eighth story – a slow start to a quick home birth

Carol had had a difficult pregnancy and was keen to go into labour. Her story continues from Part 1.

I awoke on Mother's Day with a thick, clear show. I willed labour to start, but it didn't. All that week I had more shows and, by Thursday, they had become bloody. Also on Thursday I noticed my Braxton Hicks pains had become frequent and regular (every five minutes, lasting thirty seconds), but not painful.

After one and a half days of this (some of the pains were even disturbing my sleep), I was incredibly unhappy when my labour still hadn't started. I rang my midwife, Cathy, and asked her to please come and see if these niggly pre-labour pains were opening my cervix at all.

I was 2.5 to 3 centimetres dilated and the head four-fifths descended. After an hour and a half I was further dilated and the head was lower down, but I just knew this wasn't labour, so I sent Cathy home.

It was now 7 pm and 21-month-old James's bedtime. Since I was still breastfeeding my toddler, I nursed him to sleep, hoping to trigger stronger contractions. I did indeed bring on stronger, longer pains, and did dilate to 4 centimetres. However, it wasn't time for this baby yet, and everything just stopped until Saturday the next day.

My due date, 16 May, arrived. At about lunchtime I started feeling odd and unable to cope. I was alone with six of our seven children and I needed someone with me. Then, all of a sudden, I felt contractions and a bit of a pushing sensation. Too scared to go to the toilet in case the baby was there, I went to the phone and tried to contact someone. I couldn't get hold of my midwife. Neither could I get hold of my husband, and my support person lived too far away. I needed someone urgently (or so I thought), so I rang my neighbour, Kim, who was home and came straight over. Eventually I got hold of everyone else and had a house full of people when we realised it was a false alarm.

Feeling very let down and having now given up on the birth of my baby, I went to bed at 9 pm with a heavy heart. I couldn't wait to have my baby, and it just wasn't happening. I don't even remember falling asleep, but all of a sudden I was awake having heard a small pop. I also thought I was leaking something. (I didn't at that time realise how much I had saturated the mattress!) Since my waters had never properly broken with my other children, this was a totally new experience.

Clem saw me and quickly sent our children to bed before they realised what was happening. I made it to the toilet, where the pains started. This was the real thing. It was just after 11 pm – less than one hour before midnight. Now lasting at least one minute, these pains were excruciating for about ten seconds during their peak.

Pretty soon, Clem came to see what was happening.

'Quick, call Cathy,' I told him. 'I think my waters have broken, and these contractions are very painful. I think you had better call Mary as well.' Clem was of two minds. First, he was scared it would happen too fast and he would have to deliver the baby himself. 'I want you in the hospital,' he said. Then, the next minute, he wouldn't call Mary until Cathy had arrived and checked me – 'Just to make sure it wasn't another false alarm.'

Approximately half an hour later, Cathy arrived. I hadn't been able to move from the toilet seat, as the pains were too frequent and severe, so Cathy now helped me through to the bedroom. Here she pronounced me 5.5 centimetres dilated and going to have this baby. Clem then called Mary (a 45-minute drive away), but she didn't make it. About ten minutes later, I was 7 centimetres dilated, in terrible pain and wanting to push.

Since making it to the bedroom I had managed to stay upright for the contractions, and had hung onto and hugged Cathy when I needed to. Clem also supported me with his presence, but now I had to sit down. I even wanted to lie down, but when I did the contractions became totally unbearable, so I quickly got Cathy to help me upright again.

By now I was pushing and sitting upright on the edge of my bed. The pushing sensation was delightful, as it took away the pain of the contractions, and I could feel the head coming out.

When I realised it was actually happening I lifted my bottom slightly off the bed so I wouldn't push the baby's head into the mattress. Being in this position (sitting upright with bottom slightly raised), I actually saw my baby coming out. What an incredible sight that was – and not painful at all. But Cathy did make me stop pushing once the head was out, as the cord was loosely around the baby's neck. Cathy removed the cord from the baby's neck (which did hurt a bit), then let me push the baby through the cord.

It was 12.24 am on Sunday, 17 May. I had delivered following a labour lasting just one hour and 24 minutes. The immediate high I felt was incredible, and the tremendous love I felt for my baby, who we named Christine, was just amazing. Her Apgar scores were 9 and 9, and she was my biggest baby yet, just less than 3600 grams. Even more amazing, this was the first time I hadn't torn, and the first time I had been upright for second-stage labour – I normally get stuck in a lying down position.

Cathy, who works in a maternity hospital where she is a midwife, as well as caring for women who have home births, told me that if I had been having the baby in hospital they would definitely have induced me because of my two false alarms, and would probably have given me Syntocinon to speed up delivery of the placenta, because of my age (35) and number of previous children. As it was, Christine was immediately put to my breast, even before I had delivered the placenta. The cord was left unclamped and uncut until it had stopped pulsating, something that couldn't have been done had I been given Syntocinon. The placenta came out about ten minutes after I delivered Christine. By putting your baby to the breast, natural contractions cause this to happen quickly anyway.

Thinking about my baby filled me with great joy. How grateful I was to have another precious bundle. Nothing can compare to the wonderful sight of excited older children as they one by one awaken and view their new sibling for the first time. In fact, the whole family had had a joyful experience because I had given birth at home to our eighth baby. Mummy was still at home and hadn't disappeared in the middle of the night, older breastfed toddlers could still cuddle up and nurse with their new sister, and jealousy and 'separation-from-Mum worry' hadn't occurred.

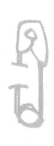

Strategies for minimising pain during labour

- Try not to go to the hospital or birth centre until you are in established labour, as you may become discouraged if you are sent home. But don't leave it too late if this is not your first baby and you know that your labours are quick.

- Try to avoid labouring in the presence of people you were not planning to be there, as this may cause you to become inhibited and consequently depressed or disheartened.

- Be prepared for at least 60 seconds of pain with each contraction, and try to find something to focus on to take your mind off the pain:

  – count down the contraction with a clock that has a second hand

  – gaze into a friend's eyes

  – have a friend put pressure on the area where you are feeling the pain

  – press a hot-water bottle/hot pack into the area of pain.

- Keep your bladder empty while you are in labour, as a full bladder can slow down your labour by putting added pressure on your cervix.

- Do not have too high an expectation as to what distraction can do to minimise the pain. It will help, but it will not remove the pain. Many women opt for the drug pethidine, thinking it will remove the pain altogether. It will not do this and will normally put you to sleep between contractions, forcing you to wake up to a new contraction each time. As a consequence, where the contractions were once painful, but coming after a minute's break, it may now seem as if you are experiencing one long, continuous pain with no time to prepare for it.

- Expect that in the course of your labour you will eventually have very painful contractions, but that they will pass and you will have a break between this one and the next (even if it is only a one-minute break).

- Remember that if your contractions are close together (coming every two minutes), your baby's birth may not be far away.

- Try to imagine the contractions bringing your baby down the birth canal and closer to being born and in your arms.

- Try to remain upright as much as possible. While you are flat on your back, your body has to work harder to contract efficiently, and the resulting contractions can be more painful.

- Go with your body and do what you feel is helpful. Every woman is different, so different things will help different people. Adopt the positions that best suit you. For example, if you feel like leaning forward into a beanbag, or pushing onto a chair, do so. If you feel like walking around or keeping still, do so.

- Try to avoid being told what to do if your body is telling you otherwise. For example, lying flat on your back for an examination may increase the pain of your contractions, so get someone to help you back into an upright position once your examination is over, rather than stay in this position. Write a birth plan in advance stating that you wish to remain upright for as long as possible.

- If the different positions and methods you try do not help you cope and you opt for pain relief, do not feel as though you have failed. Giving birth is not a competition to see who can do it best. It is your own personal experience, with the main aim being to produce a live, healthy baby!

- The use of heat is often a helpful way to reduce discomfort, and many women prefer to spend most of their labour in the shower or bath. Try getting into a shower and running hot water over the area that hurts.
- Try giving birth on a birth stool, as you are upright and being aided by the force of gravity, enabling the second stage of labour to be faster and easier. While you are on the birth stool, you are also keeping your weight off your sacrum and lessening the pain of your contractions.
- As the baby's head emerges, stop pushing either by panting or blowing. This facilitates a slow birth of the baby's head, which reduces the risk of your perineum tearing. Try to listen to the instructions. The midwife or doctor's may place a hand on the baby's head to help control the speed with which it emerges. This helps the perineum stretch gradually. Write a birth plan stating that this is what you want to happen, if possible.
- Try giving birth in the squatting position, as here your sacrum becomes free and actually moves back to widen the pelvic outlet, especially if your top half is leaning forward.

Karen's birth story

When I had my ultrasound I found out the baby's sex, but my husband, Ricc, didn't want to know. I felt as though I had a secret and intimate connection with the baby. My husband called him Yoda, as he thought that's who the baby looked like in the ultrasound pictures.

I was disappointed when my due date came and went without incident. The baby's head had engaged early, so I assumed he was ready to arrive. A few days later I woke at 4 am to an uncomfortable cramping feeling across my abdomen. I knew labour was starting and felt anxious and excited. My husband was asleep and I didn't want to wake him, so I dozed for the next few hours. By then the pain kept waking me and I was too excited to sleep. I got up and showered and started cleaning and washing clothes. I couldn't sit down and instinctively walked around, and when I had a contraction I would stand and breathe through it. The pain was bearable and I continued to potter around.

By 11 am the contractions were becoming more painful. All I could think about was how uncomfortable the car trip to the hospital was going to be. If we left it much longer, I wouldn't be able to bear it. I also had a grave fear of not arriving in time and having to deliver at home or in the car (despite the fact that I am a nurse and my husband is a doctor).

When we arrived at the hospital and checked in, we made our way to the unit. My blood pressure was taken and a trainee doctor took my medical history and examined me. I was already 5 centimetres dilated. It all seemed a bit surreal.

By the time my friend and support person Jacinta arrived, I was concentrating so much on my contractions I was not aware of what was happening around me. The pain had got to a point where I couldn't walk around anymore. The midwives were monitoring my baby's heart and I was sucking madly on entonox [laughing gas].

I didn't want comfort, I didn't want to be touched. I needed to concentrate, eyes closed, sucking the entonox. I needed to internalise everything, which was my way of staying in control. By 2.30 pm the contractions were making my whole body shake. I had an urge to bear down but knew I had to fight it because I wasn't dilated enough. The midwives were reassuring and told me that it wouldn't be long.

Just when I was feeling completely out of control and that I had to push, I got the green light to go ahead. This was the moment I had been waiting for. I got into a kneeling position with my buttocks facing the midwife and my upper body supported by pillows. I started pushing and, to my shock, also began to make strange, deep guttural sounds. One of the midwives told me to try to focus my energy on pushing instead of on the noise I was making. Once I did that, the pushing was much more efficient. I pushed for nearly an hour, which was physically exhausting. I wasn't aware of the pain as much now, as I knew there would be an end result soon.

Finally my son arrived and was put between my legs. The cord had been around his neck, so there had been a delay to remove that once the baby's head had emerged. I noticed he looked a bit flaccid and that his colour wasn't right. The midwives and my husband gave him oxygen and stimulated him to wake up. I felt very calm and knew he would be all right. My husband brought him back to me, but I was anxious for him to be looked after properly. He was taken to intensive care, for observation overnight, but I was able to visit and breastfeed him.

When my obstetrician examined me I had a very small first-degree tear, which healed on its own very quickly. After the birth I was on such a high and was so happy and excited, I felt that I could run a marathon. I had a gorgeous son who weighed 3500 grams and was 52 centimetres long. They say you forget all the pain of the delivery. I don't think you forget it, but you realise when you put it in perspective that it was all worth it.

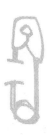

Panting

Panting in short, quick breaths is a form of breathing sometimes encouraged during second-stage labour to prevent the woman from pushing while her baby is being born.

Pushing sometimes needs to be avoided for the baby's safety. For example, if the cord is firmly wrapped around the baby's neck, it needs to be cut and tied before the head is born. Not pushing will slow the baby's delivery. A less speedy delivery is also sometimes necessary to prevent the perineum tearing and thus avoiding the need for stitches afterwards. The woman may be encouraged to pant instead of push so that the head is delivered slowly and the perineum is given a chance to stretch and better accommodate the emerging baby.

Janice's birth story

Janice suffered pneumonia and a severe dog bite during her pregnancy. Her story continues here from Part 1.

It was forty weeks exactly when I awoke at 12.45 thinking Mal must have kicked me. I was very shocked and thought he should have been more careful. The pain I felt was in the side of my stomach, but it wasn't until I was fully awake that it dawned on me that labour had now started. 'Oh no,' I thought. 'It's happening!'

Going to the bathroom, I found nothing had changed, so thought I must have imagined things. I began heading back to bed when it happened again. It was not a strong pain, more like wind, but strong enough to make me stop and think. Looking at the clock I realised this second pain had happened only five minutes since the first. I stood in the lounge room for about fifteen minutes experiencing pains which came every five minutes. I then went back to the bedroom, where I experienced a blood-stained show of mucus. I wondered if I should wake up Mal. Part of me felt silly, as I wasn't certain I was in labour and didn't want to make a fuss. But the other half was certain something was happening and began to feel scared. (I had been waiting all this time to have our baby, but now it was happening I didn't want it to go any further.) I decided to wake Mal, who was really good once he awoke, but was hard to stir in the first place.

Now the pains were getting stronger but also further apart. They were coming every eight minutes instead of five. I had so many mixed feelings. I was scared, excited, horrified and happy all rolled into one. Mal rang the hospital and explained to the midwife what I had told him, and she told us to come in.

At the hospital my contractions were timed and my blood pressure was taken, along with other routine procedures, including filling in forms. The contractions were four minutes apart, lasting thirty to forty seconds, and I thought, 'If they stay like this I can cope.' But somehow I knew they wouldn't. Instinctively I knew I should relax and not fight them. So instead of fighting the pain I just went along with it.

As time passed the contractions became stronger and stronger and closer together, but I was still managing to relax. Time seemed to be passing quickly, and before I knew it, it was 7 am. My support person, Sharon, had to leave now, but she intended to get back as quickly as she could. Also at this time I was given an injection of pethidine, which I later regretted. (I don't believe the pethidine stopped the pain. It just made me feel weird and less in control. It slowed my thinking and made it harder for me to concentrate on handling the pain. I would not take pethidine with future pregnancies.)

Now that Sharon had gone, Mal, who had fallen asleep on the floor, woke up and began encouraging me. His timing was perfect, as I needed him very much. Unfortunately Sharon came back too late to actually witness the birth, but did the next best thing by coming to see our brand new baby.

The midwife who had met us at the door was lovely but also due to finish her shift at 7 am. She was disappointed I was not going to have the baby on her shift. 'Now I'll be thinking about you all day,' she said. 'But if you like I can give you an examination to see how far dilated you are.'

The examination didn't hurt and I was discovered to be 3.5 centimetres dilated. I was happy to hear that but had hoped I was further along. Shortly after the examination I felt my waters break. At the same time my baby moved down and blocked off the gap, meaning that my membranes were unable to rupture completely. A midwife later said that my baby would probably have been born sooner if my waters had broken properly at this time.

By 10 am the pethidine had worn off. One and a half hours later I was taken to the labour ward in a wheelchair, which I hated. This turned out to be the worst part of my labour, as I had to sit on my bottom with every pain (which seemed to intensify them). The midwife then asked if I felt like pushing, but I didn't.

Once in the labour ward I was put onto a bed and examined. I was now 8.5 centimetres dilated. The midwife once again asked if I wanted to push, but I still didn't have any urges. She later asked me a third time, probably because my contractions were very strong and close together. In the meantime I was almost wrecking the bed, grabbing hold of the bars behind me as the pains began getting on top of me. I had planned to give birth in an upright position, as I thought the force of gravity would aid my delivery and make it easier, but when the time came I was in fact lying on my side with one leg pushed against Mal, as I was too exhausted to coordinate standing with the pains.

My doctor arrived and straight away asked if I had been examined. The midwife had done a second examination and found me fully dilated, but since I had had no urges to push, the doctor felt I may not be, so wanted to examine me again. But then I gave this almighty involuntary grunt and he quickly changed his mind, instead telling me to push. I still didn't feel like pushing, but everyone was coaching me to do so, so I did. All the while I felt I was pushing against something immovable.

The doctor now told me to push into the lower half of my body, not the top, but I found it very hard to listen to him. When I finally got the hang of it I began feeling disheartened because I couldn't feel the baby coming down. I started to believe it wasn't working. Soon the doctor was telling me to push with every contraction. It was hard but I kept myself going, thinking, 'It's almost over.' I was pushing so hard, Mal later told me he thought my jugular vein was going to burst.

I asked my doctor, 'Why isn't he coming?' to which he replied, 'I don't know.' Then all of a sudden the baby's head started to appear.

'Soon I'm going to ask you to stop pushing,' my doctor said.

'What, why?' were my immediate thoughts. 'Just when I've gotten the hang of this!' And then he did tell me to stop, asking me to pant instead. I didn't know how to pant and the doctor had to show me. I was really only panting a matter of seconds but it felt like an eternity, as I couldn't get enough breath while doing so. I wanted to stop but the doctor was saying, 'Just a little more, don't stop yet.'

Our baby was slowly emerging with every pant. He was coming out in little spurts, just like a jackhammer. It was an awesome sight, Mal later told me. Then suddenly our baby's head and shoulders were right out while I was still only panting. The doctor now told me to push, which I did, and finally, at long last, our baby was out. I gave a big sigh of relief, followed quickly by, 'How big is he?'

As it turned out, Dylan weighed 2960g and was 48 centimetres. I was most surprised, since I had been expecting a 5 kilogram baby following that earlier antenatal appointment. They now took our baby away to be checked, but I could still see what was happening, as they kept him in the same room. The midwife then gave me an injection to bring on my placenta. I noticed it was rushed away as soon as it came out. I was never told of any problems so presumed nothing had been wrong.

During my delivery I didn't tear, thanks to my doctor who made me stop pushing at that crucial moment when our baby's head crowned. The baby had been born covered in dried meconium. It was in his eyes and ears, as well as the rim of his nose. It actually took several days and several scrubs to completely remove, and poor Dylan came to hate his baths. (Although he did later learn to enjoy them.) Apparently we were fortunate our baby hadn't taken the meconium into his lungs. He was healthy at birth and there were no long-term repercussions.

Avoiding a difficult second stage

Some women experience problems when it comes to pushing their baby out. This can happen if they are fully dilated but do not feel the urge to push.

When pushing without an urge, you are more likely to tear, as your tissues have not had a chance to thin and fan out. It can also rob you of that wonderful sensation you feel when pushing with your natural urges.

Alternatively, you may feel like pushing but not be fully dilated. Pushing before full dilation can cause damage and swelling to the cervix and also delay the birth.

In her book *New Active Birth*, Janet Balaskas recommends you do not rush the second stage, encouraging the mother to take time and follow her instincts.

Kuini's first birth story

Kuini had planned a home birth for her first child. Her story continues from Part 2.

It was very early on a Saturday morning when my contractions started. Once Patrick, my partner, had awoken, we phoned Joan, who told us to call her when my contractions were coming two to three minutes apart. She commented that birthing was basically about waiting for things to take their natural course. Since my contractions were coming about twenty minutes apart, we decided to visit my cousin. My cousin has a property with lots of lovely, big pine trees, and I had an urge to be near trees and greenery. We stayed there all day eating and laughing.

Patrick and I now raced home, where Patrick cooked a lovely meal. We now decided to do some housework, because the midwife was coming over. We didn't finish it until midnight. By this time my contractions were coming every ten minutes and lasting a minute in length. There was no pain – just a feeling of movement and tightening across my stomach. But I knew they were contractions because of the regular manner in which they were coming.

I had contractions all through the night. I went to the toilet and emptied my bowels a lot, but by 3 am felt so scared and lonely that I vomited out of fear. I decided to go back to bed and note how long my contractions lasted and how long it was between each one. They were one minute long, coming every three minutes. At 8 am we decided to phone our midwife, who said to phone her back when the contractions were one minute apart. (She later told me that first-timers usually have a long labour.) So, Pat decided to bake some cookies and make some soup for visitors and the midwife.

Joan arrived at about 2 pm. We hadn't phoned her; she had simply decided that by 2 o'clock my contractions would be about one minute apart, and she was right. It was now that Joan gave me my first vaginal examination. My cervix was dilating well and was very soft, but my waters hadn't broken yet. At this point I was on a natural high and only wanted my cats in the bedroom with me, so Joan and Pat decided to have lunch in the dining room. The cats made me feel peaceful, happy and safe. Pat tried to chase them out because he thought they had too many germs, but Joan insisted that if this was what I wanted then we should leave my 'security blanket' cats in there. I really felt these cats were like my anaesthetic.

Then my sister Liz arrived with her husband John and my nieces Niki and Melissa. It was about 4 pm and Joan was giving me another examination to see how far dilated my cervix was. My sister wanted her little girls (aged eight and nine) to look at my vagina during the examination. Poor little things didn't want to, and neither did I. Joan sensed my distress and so did Liz's husband, John. He tried to ask my sister to leave everything alone and suggest that it might be better if they left, but Liz now started talking loudly at me, saying, 'It's okay, isn't it? It's okay?' She was very angry and, because of my vulnerable state, I just couldn't handle it, so I got up and left the room. I had to go somewhere nice and peaceful outside.

While outside, I started to squat and enjoy the reassuring warmth of the sun. I didn't want to deal with other people's dramas. I just wanted to give birth.

My sister came outside and stood between the sun and me. 'What's the matter with you?' she said.

Joan came and asked her to leave. (Joan later told me she could see how distressed I was becoming, and her job was to maintain a smooth and peaceful birth.) I was very upset and began hyperventilating, so Joan got me back into bed. Because I was distressed, my contractions became painful, my blood pressure skyrocketed and my cervix closed 2 centimetres. Joan commented that a woman under stress will not have a soft cervix which dilates gently, but her cervix can remain fixed and hard, and, as in my case, can actually close back up. Joan now gave me some homoeopathic rescue remedy and acupuncture (which I hated), and she and Pat left me alone for two hours so I could calm down.

At around 6 pm, Joan and Pat came back into the room. My contractions were about twenty seconds apart and I was fully dilated. At this point, although in no pain, I had no urge to push and was sort of bored, just wanting to get it over and done with. Pat hopped onto the bed and started to hold my hand and hug me. The only pain I felt was Pat crushing my hand. I wanted to tell him to go away, but I didn't want to hurt him. Eventually we bonded and he was extremely emotionally and physically supportive. In fact, he turned out to be better than the cats!

Going through transition, I became irritated with Joan and tersely asked of her, 'And how many children have you had?'

'Five,' she calmly replied. That shut me up.

My waters still hadn't broken, so Joan asked me if I wanted to give birth to the baby with membranes intact or did I want her to cut them. I asked which was the painful one and she said 'neither'. So we decided to cut the membranes. Joan consequently cut them so gently I could hardly even feel it.

A slight dribbling of fluid followed, which quickly turned into gushing once Joan pressed down on my uterus. I was now in the squatting position, leaning forward on my hands and bearing down. Pat had his face right under my vagina, giving me reports that he could see the baby's head while I was bearing down. He became very excited and this was encouraging me. At this point, Joan decided to phone the doctor because I was beginning to crown.

The doctor arrived only to discover that Joan and Pat were taking care of everything. The atmosphere was highly charged but harmonious. He said he didn't have a job to do, so subsequently got to take the photographs.

It felt wonderful when the baby's head crowned, and I was actually in ecstasy when the baby's head came out so smoothly. To be truthful, it was just like an orgasm. Then, when the baby's body was born, it was pleasurable.

Julia came out. Joan gently lifted her onto my stomach and she got straight up onto her forearms and looked around. She didn't cry. I was absolutely stunned at this complete, separate human being and thought, who is this?

Soon our baby called out and I responded saying, 'Come here, darling.' She crawled up onto my stomach and clamped onto my breast. She then suckled for dear life. Once again I was stunned.

Baby Julia and I now cuddled and kissed. Pat's face was shining like a light and he looked just like a mother hen.

Julia weighed 3458 grams and was 55 centimetres in length. She was born at 7.35 pm after a 40-hour, virtually painless labour.

At about 3 am I awoke to find this baby clamped onto my breast once again. I was amazed and delighted. We then had a special time together in the wee hours of the morning.

After Julia fell asleep, I got up, washed the dishes and sheets, then in the morning got up and made Pat a cup of tea. After all, he had had a hard night giving birth.

More points for an easier birth

It can be a big boost to your morale during labour if you have already established relationships with the people who are going to be present at your baby's birth.

Understandably, a woman often feels extremely vulnerable during this time. She needs to know that the person attending her birth cares for her and wants to be there. It can also be important to feel that you are being supported in your choices. For example, you may wish to take all your clothes off before delivery so your newborn can be placed straight onto your stomach or breast and suckle if the baby wants to. If someone present disapproves of your actions, however, you may instead become inhibited and not attempt to do this. To ensure your support people are not uncomfortable or embarrassed by your actions, discuss with them how you feel and what you may feel like doing during the course of your labour.

In some instances, you might have been able to develop relationships with the midwives who will attend your birth if you have been attending a birth centre for your antenatal care, or have employed a midwife for a home birth. More often, however, your medical attendants will be unknown to you, as is often the case in the labour ward of a busy hospital, where large numbers of staff will be working, and regular staff changeovers occur. This is why it is important for your peace of mind to bring along a support person who knows you and your plans. In this way you are preparing them for your possible behaviour and needs. When the time comes, your birth assistants will be comfortable with your actions.

Support people should keep in mind that it is the woman who is giving birth, therefore her needs and requirements should be supported. If she wants to walk around, or have a shower right up to the crowning, encourage her to do so.

Jane's second birth story

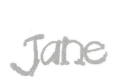

Jane had planned a water birth at home. Her story continues from Part 1.

The care I received during the pregnancy was excellent. The midwives would come to our home, which I found great because of my busy lifestyle. We discussed many issues at great length. Frank and Joshua [Jane's husband and son] were both very involved. I visited the obstetrician once as a courtesy. I liked having her as a backup, in case I needed to be transferred to hospital. She respected my decision to have a home birth and was open to different ideas for management in the case of complications.

I left work at the hospital at 34 weeks, but I continued to work at home. I had a number of large projects, which I tried in vain to complete before the baby arrived. I also continued with my home birth practice and running prenatal classes. I was worried that this baby would come early, too.

Sunday, 30 September arrived. I was nearly 39 weeks pregnant and I told myself that I had done enough – I was now ready for the baby to be born. I felt a real change in myself.

I spent time with work colleagues on Monday night. I was feeling relaxed and happy, though quite uncomfortable from the pregnancy. I went to bed on Tuesday night feeling nothing unusual. From midnight I made frequent trips to the toilet. To my surprise I awoke at 4.30 am with a contraction. I thought it must have been a strong Braxton Hicks. I got up to go to the toilet yet again and another contraction came within minutes of the other. In denial, I went back to bed, where the contractions continued to come at around three-minute intervals. I couldn't believe it. I was sure that it was all going to stop soon.

The contractions were becoming more painful and I couldn't get comfortable in bed. I had a fear that this labour was going to be fast, but then I did not want to call people too early. In a minor dilemma, I decided to call Nicole, one of my support people, at around 5.30 am. (I knew Nicole probably had work planned for that day and that if I needed her in a hurry she would have to negotiate peak-hour traffic.) I finally decided that this was probably real labour, so I asked Frank to get the birth pool ready. I rationalised that if everything stopped we could empty it.

At around 6.30 am I called Karen, my sister, who was going to be Joshua's support person. I was now convinced that the contractions were here to stay. I contacted Myra, one of my midwives, just before 7 am to let her know what was happening. She said she would have breakfast and that I should call her again when I wanted her to come. The contractions continued with good intensity. I paced up and down the house with my hot pack, not wanting anyone to touch me. Myra telephoned an hour later, asking if I needed her. I said I wasn't sure, but she said she would come over and see how things were going – she could always leave if there was not a lot happening. Myra arrived just after 8 am. I was in the shower. It was great – I had privacy, and the warm water really helped with the contractions.

The contractions were now coming every two minutes. I longed to hop into the birth pool, but I wanted to leave it until I was at least 6 centimetres dilated. I kept looking at the pool and finally thought, this is ridiculous, so hopped in. It was bliss. I felt as if I almost stopped having contractions. They were just like tightenings. During one of my trips to the toilet, I decided I needed to know if I was progressing, so I did my own internal. I estimated I was around 7 centimetres dilated and I could feel a large bag of waters in front of the baby's head. It was only 9 am; I was so pleased with my progress. The contractions picked up in intensity, but I felt totally relaxed between them.

At around 10.30 am I asked Myra to check my progress (I was actually doubting my own assessment, imagining that I was not anywhere near as advanced as I'd believed I was, as the labour wasn't that bad). Myra announced that I was 9.5 centimetres dilated (just an anterior lip left to go). I couldn't believe it. I began willing my waters to break, as in my mind, when this happened the baby would come soon after. I was starting to feel pressure in my bottom, but no urge to push.

The nature of the contractions then changed and I felt I was not coping with them anymore. I started pushing slightly with some contractions, but still really didn't have the urge. I had to constantly keep telling myself that I could do it, that it wasn't long to go. The pain was incredible, worse than I could possibly have imagined.

At 11 am my waters broke when I gave a decent push with one of the contractions. It was an amazing feeling. I felt the bag of waters come down into my vagina and then burst. I continued to breathe through the contractions. I decided about half an hour later that I would push with the contractions, as I had continual pressure in my bottom and I was sure I was fully dilated. After a short time I felt no progress was being made, so I asked Cathy, my other midwife who had arrived over an hour before, to check that the cervix had completely opened. Of course it had. I was pushing with all my might, even though I still didn't feel the urge. I kept checking for the baby's head, as I had absolutely no sense of it moving down. It was very close now, but taking a lot of effort. I was experiencing incredible back and pubis symphysitis pain. Cathy and Myra applied a hot-water bottle and hot towels to the area, which helped somewhat. I was also given homoeopathic remedies, which also helped slightly.

Once the baby's head reached the perineum, I just about leapt out of the pool. Whoever said that you experience a burning, stinging pain was making an understatement! I would describe the pain as searing, tearing and excruciating. I had to mentally overcome my reaction to this pain to give birth. Cathy applied hot towels under the water to my perineum, which helped me to relax slightly.

The baby's head emerged with agonising slowness. The pain became so intense I was unable to tell when I had a contraction. I asked Cathy to tell me when a contraction came so that I could push with it. I cannot tell you how much relief I felt once the baby's head was born. But then the most bizarre thing happened: the baby tried to pull himself back inside me a couple of times. It was a most violent movement. I knew that I was carrying a large baby, and I became concerned about birthing the baby's shoulders. I thought to myself that I should probably stand up, but the lure of the water was too strong. Myra and Frank assisted me to flex my legs backwards. I could feel Cathy trying to manoeuvre the shoulders and I pushed with all my might – Jarred's birth was difficult right up until his toes!

I can still remember the moment when I opened my eyes after giving that almighty push. There he was, my baby, under the water. I thought, 'I did it! I really did it!' The thrill of reaching for my baby and bringing him to the surface was overwhelming. There was no rush; I just held him and looked at him. It took a while before I wanted to discover his sex. He was quite pale and limp at first. I rubbed him and talked to him. The cord was still pulsating and supplying him oxygen. He gradually became nice and pink, although he remained quite floppy. He was breathing noisily, so Myra gently suctioned him and then he received some oxygen. All the while I held him and marvelled at him.

Then the contractions started again. I was quite taken aback by their intensity. I tried to push with them to birth the placenta, but it wasn't ready to come. After about twenty minutes I was concerned that Jarred's breathing was too fast and noisy. The umbilical cord had stopped pulsating, so I asked for the cord to be cut so he could be warmed up and have more attention paid to his breathing. I also felt the need to be upright. Frank cut the cord. I then kneeled, leaning on the side of the pool, and the placenta was born with the next contraction.

I was very keen at this point to get out of the pool and to dry off. A bed was made on the floor with towels and blankets, where I lay down gratefully. I needed some time out at this point, as I was feeling quite shocked from the pain of the last hour or so of the labour. I asked if they would weigh and dress Jarred for me. I soon found out why his birth had been so difficult: he weighed a decent 4300 grams. I had quite a long tear that needed stitching (Jarred's head was a good size as well). Once all this was done, I had a lovely hot shower and was then tucked up in bed with Jarred, who attached to the breast immediately and sucked contentedly.

Kuini's second birth story

The day before my labour started I had been scrubbing and cleaning everything. At about midnight that night I made the bed and lay on top of it, absolutely exhausted. At 3 am, after rolling over in bed, my waters broke and my contractions began.

After preparing the bed for the birth, I lay there through all my contractions, which were painless as they had been in my first labour, until 8 am when I phoned the midwife.

When she arrived I was found to be fully dilated. My cousin's wife came over to look after Julia, my eighteen-month-old daughter.

I had actually met my midwife, Veronica, only the day before, as my first midwife, Joan Donaley, who had delivered Julia, had had to fly to Australia for a conference. At about 9 am the doctor arrived.

As this baby was my second child, I had decided that this time around I would talk to the baby during the delivery.

'Come on, baby. Mummy's here and Mummy loves you. Help Mummy give birth to you,' I was saying to my baby.

In return, I felt my baby responding to my voice in a very encouraging way. It was definitely a two-way thing, which was very exciting.

Then, as my baby was being born, she presented her elbow first, and I remember thinking, 'Oh no, I don't want her to be pulled into the world,' but just at that moment I felt as though my whole pelvic structure collapsed for a split second, allowing my baby to pass through, arm and all!

My baby was born at 9.20 am, weighing 3684 grams. When she was born she was very tired and didn't initially want to breastfeed. It was only after everyone had left that she began to.

Over the next few days, baby Helen just slept and slept. I had to wake her up to feed her. She was such a pleasant, sweet little baby and a delight to have – and now I had two beautiful children.

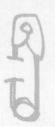

Afterpains

Afterpains are not often noticeable with the first baby. However, they frequently increase in strength with each additional birth. They feel like pre-birth contractions or period pains, and they tend to feel stronger when you are breastfeeding your baby. The pains are natural and no cause for alarm (though you should discuss any pain or discomfort that concerns you with your doctor or midwife immediately). It is common for a woman who has had four or more children to comment that her afterpains are just as painful as her labour contractions.

While in hospital, paracetemol may be offered to ease these pains. It needs to be taken half to one hour before you plan to breastfeed to be most effective. Afterpains normally start to subside by the third day after birth.

Drugs and other interventions

Everyone hopes for an easy, natural birth. However, for various reasons either during the pregnancy or during labour, medical intervention may be necessary in the birth. Medical and scientific advances have meant that unexpected events or situations that arise can be dealt with quickly and safely. For those women wanting pain relief there are now several options available, and some women may request certain interventions because they feel it is best for them.

Medical advancement has brought us to the point where it is possible to initiate labour and successfully intervene in the birth of a child. This is not to say natural is not best. For some women, though, the artificial starting of their labour, or a caesarean or forceps delivery, will improve the health of their baby or themselves, and may even be life saving. Drugs and interventions are a marvellous achievement used in their rightful place. However, sometimes there can be a tendency to overuse some procedures and put medicine over nature with little justification. This can cause a snowballing effect, with one intervention leading to another, causing unnecessary trauma for both mother and child.

This section describes some common medical interventions that can occur during labour, pain relief options, and the stories of women whose labours involved these procedures.

Induction of labour

Induction is one or more procedures that are used to artificially start labour when there is concern for the mother's or baby's health. The methods used for inducing labour are the artificial rupture of the membranes, the application of a hormonal gel near the cervix and the introduction of synthetic hormones into the bloodstream.

Prostaglandin is a hormone that helps soften the cervix. It is usually applied in a gel form near the cervix during a vaginal examination. Electronic fetal monitoring is carried out before and after the application of the gel to ensure that the baby is not in distress. A repeat dose of prostaglandin gel may be required. Some women experience nausea, vomiting or diarrhoea when it is used. If a woman's waters have broken, the prostaglandin gel is not recommended. If prostaglandin is successful, the labour that ensues is more natural than induction of labour by other methods.

Syntocinon is an artificial form of the body's natural hormone oxytocin, which causes the uterus to contract. The woman's waters are usually broken, then the Syntocinon is administered via an intravenous drip. Once the induction of labour has commenced, the rate of the drip is carefully controlled by a special pump, the dosage being gradually increased until the woman is experiencing intense, regular contractions. This is a reliable method of bringing on the labour. However, it means the mother is immobile due to the drip and monitors, and it may cause distress to the baby.

Yvette's birth story

Yvette developed PUPPP during her pregnancy. Her story continues from Part 1.

The night brought only two hours sleep – not a great rest before the arduous task of labour. The next morning it seemed very amusing to be driving off to the hospital ready for the birth with a thermos and a packed lunch for my husband. We arrived at 8 am and I was put on the monitor to check the heartbeat of the baby. A **cannula** was inserted in my wrist ready for the drip – the PUPPPs prevented them from inserting this in the back of my hand. At 9 am they ruptured my membranes and encouraged me to walk around in the hope that this would bring on labour.

My mum, who was to be one of my support people, arrived and settled in to do some embroidery while waiting. My husband also worked on his tapestry. I would have also done some embroidery but couldn't, due to the itch. We had a real little craft workshop happening there.

At 10.30 am it became obvious that labour was not going to happen spontaneously, so I was started on the Syntocinon drip. It took a while to get the dosage right to create good, strong contractions, and all the while I walked around the delivery suite trying to help things along. At 12.30 my lunch arrived, which I was surprised to be allowed to have.

Soon after lunch the contractions that I was having started to feel stronger than just period pains, and I knew that things were really beginning to happen. I was sitting on the bed and soon decided that lying down would be a much better option. My husband began to massage my lower back. The pain became stronger and I asked the midwife what we could do about some drugs. She suggested either gas or pethidine. I opted for the pethidine, and while waiting for that to start to work, I also began to use the gas. My mum and husband alternated with the duty of massaging my lower back.

Being on the gas was really very funny. It caused the weirdest sensations and made me say some very strange things. In between each contraction I would stop using the gas and begin to come out of the 'fog'. At some points I was very aware of what was happening. The monitor that had been around my stomach to record the contractions was removed at some stage, but I was able to give them a fairly accurate idea of when the next one was coming.

During the contractions, which were 30 seconds apart, I can remember thinking, 'This isn't bad enough to want an epidural.' I hadn't wanted to have an epidural but had decided to leave my options open – after all, I had never been through labour before. I didn't feel the need to scream, it seemed the farthest thing from what I felt would help me.

After what didn't seem very long I suddenly realised that I felt the need to push. In the next break between contractions I asked my mum to ask the midwife (who had temporarily left the room) if I was allowed to push yet. A midwife came in to check me and said (to my absolute surprise) that I could. I was so disbelieving that I asked three times between the next few contractions if I really was allowed to push already. I am absolutely sure that at one point during the pushing I yelled, 'I don't want an episiotomy'. I am told by my husband, though, that this never happened.

After about 30 minutes of pushing, the head emerged. Mum had said to me that you feel a tremendous amount of physical relief when the head comes out, but I wasn't even aware that it had until they told me. At this point I asked whether it was a girl or a boy. One of the midwives replied, 'You can't tell from just the head.' Very soon afterwards, Emma Joy was born. It was incredible!

Most of our friends thought I was having a boy because of the way I had been carrying Emma, so to find out that it was a girl was amazing. Apparently one of the first things I said in my happy delirium was, 'Now I can make smocked dresses.' (These things are important to us needleworkers!)

In total, the active labour had been three and a half hours. I found that there had been no chance to use any of those fancy labouring positions we had learnt of in the prenatal classes, because my contractions had been so close together that there was no time in between to even move, and I don't think I could have supported any of my body weight.

In the days following Emma's birth the rash became worse, spreading to more parts of my legs and arms. I was put on an antihistamine to reduce the inflammation and stop the itch, which made me and Emma (as I was breastfeeding) quite drowsy. A dermatologist prescribed copious amounts of a stronger steroid cream that also somewhat assisted in relieving the itch. I found going home from hospital the most effective treatment, because suddenly I was so busy I didn't have time to scratch any more. The rash slowly disappeared over the next three weeks.

We learnt from the internet that PUPPP occurs when a woman becomes allergic to her stretch marks and then breaks out in a rash. Strangely enough, it is also somehow linked to the father. Due to some sort of immunological quirk, it is very rare for PUPPP to recur in subsequent pregnancies, except if the pregnancy is a first pregnancy with a new partner. This suggests that the condition may be linked to what the father contributes to the make-up of the new baby.

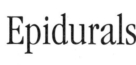

Epidurals

An epidural is an injection of local anaesthetic (some-times combined with other drugs) through a catheter into the epidural space, an area located around the spinal cord. It numbs the body from the waist down for between one and three hours. A tube is left in place so the epidural can be topped up. Epidurals take between ten and twenty minutes to put in place, and a further five to twenty minutes before the anaesthetic takes effect. The woman must stay as still as possible (the staff will help the woman to remain still) while the anaesthetist ensures the epidural is correctly positioned.

Properly administered, **epidural anaesthesia** is a very effective form of pain relief. If the epidural is allowed to wear off towards the end of the second stage of labour, the woman should be able to push her baby out; if it is still effective, the woman will find pushing difficult, as she cannot feel the contractions or her lower body. In some cases, midwives and doctors try to encourage a normal birth by watching the contractions on a monitor and telling the woman when to push.

Disadvantages

There are a number of disadvantages associated with an epidural anaesthetic. These include: increased risk of forceps birth (by three times), increased risk of caesarean birth, difficulty passing urine in labour (a catheter is inserted into the urethera to overcome this), rise in the woman's temperature (sometimes requiring intravenous antibiotics), and the epidural may not work properly. You should also be aware that 1 in 100 women develop a severe headache, 1 in 550 women have numb patches on their legs that persist for a number of months, and 1 in 4000 women experience a life-threatening emergency.

Top-ups

At some stage during an epidural, the numbing effect will wear off and the pain will return (usually about two hours after it has been administered). At this stage, the woman will be offered a top-up, with more epidural anaesthetic being injected through the fine plastic tube in place in her back if she wishes for it.

If approaching the second stage of labour, the woman may not be given a top-up, as the numbing effect may make it difficult or impossible for her to push her baby out, resulting in a forceps delivery. If labour is not imminent, however, further anaesthetic will be offered.

Susan Susan's birth story

Susan had appendicitis during her pregnancy but recovered well. Her story continues from Part 1.

Early on a Friday morning at 39 weeks, I was awoken at 3 am with mild pains coming every ten minutes. John got up also, so the two of us now sat timing these contractions, while John wrote down how often they were coming. This kept going all through the day, with the pains becoming stronger and closer together. At 11 pm we phoned the hospital to let them know we were coming in.

I was 3 centimetres dilated when we arrived at the hospital. My contractions were coming every five minutes and were so painful that I spent all night in the shower, which eased my pain a great deal. At 6 am my mother arrived and the three of us now walked around the corridors. Every time I had a contraction I would hold onto John, and the walls! By 10 am I had used the gas mask, which I didn't like at all, as the doctor didn't turn it on and I felt like I was choking. Even after he did turn it on, I didn't want it any more, as I didn't feel comfortable with it. So they now gave me pethidine, which didn't do a thing to help.

By 1 pm the midwife came and asked if I wanted to push, saying I was fully dilated. I didn't feel the urge, but since she had suggested it I thought I may as well. So, at 1.15 pm, feeling very excited and under the impression that I was about to give birth, I started to push. Some time later I was asked to stop because the baby's head had suddenly turned and was now in a bad position. I later found out this hadn't been the case.

After another examination it was discovered that I had swollen up internally and lost all my dilation. Apparently this had happened because I had been told to push too soon. I had been pushing against an incompletely dilated cervix. I was now given an epidural and my labour was induced. It was 2.30 pm. John was given a beanbag, a couple of sheets and a pillow, and we all had a wonderful rest.

A couple of hours later, when the epidural had worn off, I was fully dilated and able to start pushing again. However, my cervix was still swollen and it took another two hours for me to deliver our baby. I had pillows behind me, my mother on one side and my husband on the other, with my mother straightening my back every time I began to push. I don't know how I would have had the strength to continue if it wasn't for them doing this.

Then, at 6.30 pm, my little boy was finally born. We were all thrilled! I remember crying because my first thoughts were, 'I don't want anyone to take him away. I don't want anything to ever happen to him.'

Our little son weighed 3265 grams and was 50 centimetres long. He was completely healthy and has been a great joy to us ever since. I have since given birth to another baby boy after an uncomplicated ten-hour labour, quite different from Angelo's 33-hour labour, and I am now five months pregnant with our third child.

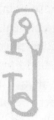

Forceps

Forceps are tong-shaped instruments used to pull the baby out of the woman's vagina when the birth has become difficult, or to turn the baby if it is facing the wrong way.

The forceps are placed on either side of the baby's head, with the doctor pulling downwards on them during a contraction. This brings the baby further down the birth canal.

If this procedure is to be performed, the woman will first be asked to lie on her back and her legs will be placed in stirrups. A local anaesthetic is injected into her perineum and an episiotomy is usually performed.

Forceps and **vacuum extraction** are used when the baby is in distress, when the baby is in a position that is making the birth difficult (forceps are used to rotate the baby into a better position), or if the woman is unable to push (due, for example, to exhaustion or a medical condition where it is considered dangerous to push).

Jo's birth story

I was 39 weeks and one day through a perfect pregnancy when I got up at 3 am on Wednesday 12 May for the familiar bladder-emptying exercise that accompanies that particular stage (and most other stages, it seems) of pregnancy. After sitting on the loo, I wasn't sure that I had produced what I had intended to. I was pretty fuzzy at 3 am, so I went back to bed and told Fred he was not allowed to flush the contents of the lavatory.

At 5.30 am I got up to 'go' again, and this time I was certain that my waters had broken, so I woke Fred (again) with the news that today we would have a baby and I began to organise the last-minute things for my hospital bag. At about 6 am the contractions started, and to begin with they were pretty easy to deal with. I started writing down the times they occurred on the back of an envelope. At about 7.30 am I rang my best pal (also my sister-in-law), whom I had promised to tell when it all started.

I rang the hospital at almost 8 am and gave them my scenario – broken waters, contractions around 10 minutes apart, not too hard to deal with. The midwife ascertained that this was our first baby and encouraged us to wait until the peak-hour traffic had died down and to come in whenever we were ready after that.

Peak hour was substantially over, and as I sat in the car while Fred got the bags, my neighbour brought over a bag filled with goodies to celebrate with (what a sweetheart, huh?).

My mother was scheduled to arrive from Tasmania two days later on the Friday. We had planned that if the baby came early I'd ring and she would see what she could do about getting there sooner. I rang her with the news of her first grandchild's imminent arrival.

We arrived at the hospital and were shown to a very mauve delivery suite where I was required (by a calm, quiet and redheaded midwife whose name now escapes me) to produce various bodily substances for testing. My blood pressure was taken, I was given a batch of enormous sanitary napkins and was assured that the doctor would be rung. We were then left to our own devices for what seemed ages. However, we learned that Mum had rearranged her flights and would be arriving at about 6.30 pm. I was sure she'd be a granny by then.

By this time I had started to get vocal, quietly groaning with each contraction. It was involuntary and it seemed to distract me from the pain or help me through the contractions, or maybe both. We set up the oil burner with lavender oil in it (very appropriate given the décor of the room). I also became rather attached to a heat pack, which I held down low against my hard-working uterus.

At about 11 am I started to feel that things were getting pretty painful, but I had resolved to get through this with no drugs. Fred offered to rub my bulging tummy; however, during contractions, I didn't want anyone to touch me. Poor husband. Here I'd been telling him for months how he had to be this great help during labour, and now I was spurning his assistance.

The redheaded midwife returned and, upon seeing the look on my face, proffered, 'The doctor has ordered you pethidine,' which, in the best traditions of self-sacrifice, I bravely refused. At this stage the contractions were less than two minutes apart, and quite painful. I decided I'd try having a shower. What a fabulous idea this turned out to be. It really made a difference to my ability to tolerate the pain. Standing in the shower with lovely warm water on my tummy, I encouraged Fred to join me. He'd just gone out to get changed when he poked his head back in the door with the bad news: 'Jo, the doctor's here ... '

I had to get out so the doctor could examine me. He pronounced me 5 centimetres dilated at 1 pm. I was pretty happy with that, fearing I might be only 1 or 2 centimetres, but I felt that with the contractions this close together and such a short break between them, I'd have a hard time coping with the pain for a further 5 centimetres of dilation. The doctor left and came back shortly. He'd been looking at my specimen results and blood pressure readings and he told me I had pre-eclampsia (which explained why I was suddenly so swollen). This swelling worsened after delivery – my poor ankles – and it took over a week to subside. The doctor's advice was that an epidural be administered, as they apparently stabilise blood pressure, and the baby's delivery would be instrumental (forceps), because the doctor didn't want me to push out the baby myself due to the danger of fitting and stroke with pre-eclampsia.

I was surprised and disappointed, and the doctor was really sympathetic but fairly insistent that this was the best course of action. Pooof! Out the window went all my notions of natural childbirth, and my hopes for a drug-free delivery. After a brief counsel with my husband, we then said to the doctor to do what he thought was best. Then I asked the doctor how long it would be before I had the epidural, because if I had no choice about having pain relief, I'd really like it *now*.

After twenty (long) minutes, the anaesthetist arrived. The doctor was prepping my back, and I was not really sure what was happening, so I was keeping really still when my fondest desire was to stretch out with the pain. The doctor administered the medication and slipped out of the room. I can't remember the particular order of events, but somewhere in there they also organised a catheter and a drip of magnesium sulphate (now I was hooked up to the machine that goes 'ping'). About five minutes later it was as though a heavy, dark curtain was lifted as the pain suddenly disappeared, and this grumpy, heaving, moaning person, became merely a bloated, rosy, beaming, relaxed person.

They hooked me up to a fetal monitor and we could hear the baby's heartbeat (which was reassuring under the circumstances) and 'see' the baby's movements. We could also 'see' when I was having contractions. This was interesting, as with the epidural working I had no idea. This was my first-ever experience of anaesthesia of any description whatsoever – those drugs really work! But I was also no longer an active participant in these events. I was just waiting now. To my mind I had become a passive receiver of care and instruction about this baby's birth. I now needed much more care – I had become a patient. After the epidural was administered, my contractions slowed. I was obviously now restricted to lying on a bed and could no longer take advantage of walking or being upright to help my cervix dilate and progress the labour.

There was a change of shift, and Maryka, a midwife with lots of life, came on duty. There was no pain; in fact, it was getting to be something of an anticlimax at this point. Late in the afternoon, an examination revealed that dilation had stalled at eight centimetres for some time, so they administered Syntocinon to try to hurry me along a bit. This baby was supposed to be born by now (by my reckoning), and even though I was in no pain, the medicos were worried about how tired I was. They kept telling me, 'Even though you can't feel it, you're still doing lots of work.' Not that I'm superstitious, but I wanted this baby to be born on the twelfth, and now I began to worry that it might be the thirteenth before the big event finally occurred.

Unbelievably, Mum rolls up, in person, in the delivery suite – can you believe it? All that travel and I haven't even given birth yet! That wasn't supposed to happen. It's after 8 pm and 13 May is looming large. So we take a few photos to relieve the boredom, and Fred sleeps even more – after all, my mother's here now, and he doesn't have to be totally responsible.

The shift changes again, and the latest midwife's name is Jo. She's very quiet and unobtrusive and very nice. Finally, the doctor arrives again, has a look and, what a surprise, I'm fully dilated. So now he tells me to push. What? I thought there wasn't going to be any pushing. Just a little bit of pushing and we'll see what happens. So what do I do? Just put your chin on your chest and push really hard down into your bottom, Jo tells me. Now this is the weirdest thing in the world. I'm lying there, barely even able to move my legs, feeling nothing from the waist down, and they say push into your bottom. So I do, but it's so weird and I'm going really red in the face, and they're yelling, 'Push!' and I am. But talk about dissatisfied. I can't feel a thing. I can't tell what's going on and I feel as though my face is going to blow off the front of my head.

Anyway, I'm instructed to stop pushing and the doctor says, 'You can see the head.' So then Fred has a look, and Mum does too, and I ask if there's any hair on the head – apparently there is. Now it's getting interesting. There's another brief lull in proceedings before the doctor says that it's time to get this baby out and bring out the forceps. My mother gathers herself together and begins to head for the door, aware that Fred and I want to witness the birth of our first child with just the two of us (plus the now-necessary medical staff).

'How long now?' we ask and are stunned with the reply: 'About 5 minutes – as soon as we get the room organised and another good contraction happens.' At this moment the mauve, cosy, homey delivery suite is amazingly transformed in a matter of moments to something more closely resembling an operating theatre. Out come the stirrups (from who knows where?), the bottom of the bed disappears, a bright light is pointed right up my rear end and the clinking of various metallic instruments is heard. I suggest Fred might want a chair behind him, in case it all gets kind of yukky.

The doctor is performing an episiotomy (at this point I must admit that I loved that epidural). Then the forceps are positioned around our unborn child's head – first one is inserted, then the other, then they're hooked together. The midwife is advising the doctor that, according to the fetal monitor, a contraction is beginning. I'm watching Fred. First, the doctor has to turn the baby by the head so that it is oriented the correct way to come through the birth canal. Then, once the child is facing the right way, with the next contraction the doctor braces himself and begins pulling this little baby from within me.

Fortunately I wasn't watching much (I was worried about Fred and I kept a watchful eye on him). Fred tells me that the stocky young doctor's forearms are bulging with the effort of pulling out the baby. I think the baby's head emerges at this point. The contraction stops and so does the doctor, then another one comes on and the doctor begins wrenching the poor baby out again, and out comes the baby. How amazing! I see the baby lifted in the doctor's arms – and it doesn't look too bad, not too much gunk on it and not too purple either.

Wow, a baby. I did it. The baby cries – fantastic. It's alive. I look at Fred, whose gaze seems to be stuck on the baby, and despite him telling me that he didn't want to when the time came, the doctor convinces him to cut the cord. I'm relieved and smiling – it's all over. I can relax, phew!

'Do you want to know what you've got?' the doctor asks me. The doctor points the baby at me, rear end first, and it's evident we have a son. 'What's his name?' the doctor asks. 'Nicholas Henry Charles,' I answer. He is placed in my arms and his little face is pretty angry looking – his bottom lip is tucked under and he's frowning a lot. A baby – unbelievable. He looks perfect. I am soooo clever. A tiny human that we made ourselves. We are quite stunned.

I eventually glance at the clock and am relieved to see it's 11.35 pm on the 12 May, still. Nicholas arrived at 11.25 pm weighing 3830 grams and was 51 centimetres long, with a head circumference of 36 centimetres. His Apgar scores were 9 and 10. He was put to the breast and, to my delight, latched and sucked enthusiastically.

The doctor spent ages stitching me up, as the episiotomy had been further ripped during the delivery. I lost a litre of blood from the episiotomy and tear, and was threatened with a transfusion, but thankfully a blood test revealed it would be unnecessary.

Unfortunately I wasn't allowed to get out of bed for over twelve hours, but I kept a steady eye on my sleeping, frowning little bundle. We were both exhausted, but I didn't sleep. I kept looking at him – looking at every detail of his face until it was imprinted on my brain – my beautiful son.

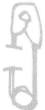

Vacuum extraction (ventouse)

A vacuum extraction is used as an alternative to a forceps birth. Vacuum extraction causes less trauma to the mother and her baby. However, forceps births are more common in Australia due to the training that doctors receive. In a vacuum extraction, the mother is usually placed on her back with her feet in stirrups and a suction cup is applied to the baby's head. A vacuum is created so the cup does not fall off, and the doctor uses traction while the mother pushes to draw the baby down the birth canal. The suction cup can be applied prior to full dilation of the cervix if this is deemed necessary. Episiotomies are not routinely performed for this procedure. Vacuum extraction can cause a lump on the baby's head that may take some time to go away.

Carmen Carmen's birth story

At an earlier visit, my doctor had reached the conclusion that my baby was getting big. I am only 122 centimetres tall. 'I think we'll have to induce you, Carmen,' he said, after informing me that I was already 2 centimetres dilated.

The induction was set for my due date, which pleased me a great deal. I was sick and tired of this painful tight feeling from the skin on my stomach being stretched to its limit. And these niggly pains were becoming quite strong, and were accompanied by back pain.

B-Day arrived and later that evening I was admitted into hospital. Shortly after my arrival, a fetal monitor was strapped across my stomach and left for half an hour to measure the contractions. I could also hear the baby's heartbeat. At 9.30 pm, a special gel was inserted to ripen my cervix and hopefully start stronger contractions. At the same time, I was given a couple of sleeping tablets.

Not long after having the gel, my pains did become stronger. I was also experiencing a lot of pressure, from the baby's head being low, and back pain. I couldn't get comfortable and spent the night pacing up and down the floors. I tried using a heat pad, which helped such a lot I found myself getting hungry, but I knew I shouldn't eat in case of trouble later.

By 6.30 am I was checked to see how far my cervix had opened. It hadn't – I was still only 2 centimetres dilated. It was then decided that I needed a drip, which was inserted almost immediately, and my waters were broken. It was horrible. The gel had given me an infection and the doctor had to apologise.

Twenty minutes later, at 7 am, I tried to phone my husband, Paul, to ask him to hurry in. I was leaking water and having to use these horrible big hospital pads. I turned around to see him standing there. Then all of a sudden I had a huge contraction, which gave me quite a fright. It was a good thing Paul was there because he helped me focus on what I was doing and began panting through the pain with me. I had to keep going to the toilet, as my membranes were constantly leaking.

My contractions were now coming every five minutes. I tried to keep my mind off them (with Paul's help), but they were so painful I had to try something else. Getting up, I walked around the corner, but it did nothing to ease the pain. Back in the induction ward, I found the pain easier to handle by holding onto the arm of the chair I was sitting in.

At 2.30 pm I was checked to see how far dilated I was. I was still only 4 centimetres, which made me a bit depressed. A midwife came and asked if I would like some pethidine. 'No,' I said, but my husband insisted.

After the pethidine injection I was able to relax, but it didn't take the pain away. The contractions were still very painful, but I continued to cope with them until 6 pm, when I was taken up to the birthing suite. But here I could hear another woman screaming. If that wasn't bad enough, it was discovered I had only dilated 1 centimetre since my last examination three and a half hours ago. It seemed like such a lot of wasted energy.

Noticing I had become distressed, the midwives offered me an epidural. I was just so disheartened I didn't care anymore, so agreed to the epidural. After inserting the epidural, the doctor left me on the operating bed, saying this was a good place to deliver my baby. A monitor was placed on my stomach to listen to the baby's heartbeat. Soon I was feeling tired and relaxed and kept drifting in and out of sleep.

At about 9.30 pm I was told that if I had dilated enough I might not need a top-up of the epidural, but I was found to be only 8 centimetres when checked. Being scared of the unknown and too frightened to feel any more pain, I was very relieved when the doctor decided to give me a top-up.

At around 11 pm it was discovered I had developed a temperature. I heard a midwife saying, 'She's getting distressed, and the baby is distressed also.' So my doctor was called back. An emergency caesarean team was on stand-by, so I was very relieved when his examination showed that I was 10 centimetres dilated, but because our baby was distressed, it had to be delivered now. The doctor gave me an episiotomy, then put a suction cap onto the baby's head to try to pull him out. But our baby kept slipping back and his shoulder was stuck. The doctor finally decided to use forceps to pull him out. I could feel the actual tugging, but because of the epidural could feel no pain. I was relieved to know our baby was finally going to be born.

James was born at 12.02 am after an eighteen-hour labour, and was very well worth it. I felt surprised at his big size, but concerned at how silent and floppy he was. My ultimate dream was to lie him on my breast and feed him straight away, but instead he had to be rushed to intensive care.

I made Paul go and check on our baby and, while he was gone, could hear another birth happening next door. My doctor came back to stitch me up, followed by Paul, who told me our baby was all right. He was breathing, but had needed oxygen, and was badly bruised as the forceps had caught him around his eye and ear. The only disheartening thing was that I wasn't able to feed my baby or hold him until the fourth day and, before this, had to express my milk into a bottle.

My first thought upon seeing him was how hairy he looked. He had hair all over his arms, legs and back, and a thick crop of jet-black hair on his head. He looked like a combination of an Eskimo and a monkey, and was just enormous. He looked very muscular and long, and I felt very proud. He was the biggest baby there, weighing 3856 grams. I remember feeling ecstatic, thinking, I'm a mummy, I'm a mummy!

Episiotomy

An episiotomy is a surgical cut made with scissors into the tissue of the perineum (the area between the vagina and anus) to enlarge the birth opening through which the baby passes. It is performed under local anaesthetic just as the baby's head crowns. An episiotomy may be done if the baby is in distress, for a forceps birth or if an extremely bad tear is anticipated. For some obstetric staff an episiotomy is a routine procedure. However, research shows that routine episiotomy should not be done. If restricted use of episiotomy is practised, women experience less perineal damage overall. Episiotomies can cause excessive blood loss, infection and haematoma formation (swelling that contains clotted blood). Women who have an episiotomy are more likely to experience a third-degree tear (this is where the episiotomy extends to the anus) with subsequent births.

Episiotomies tend to be more painful than a tear and take longer to heal. Those that advocate the liberal use of episiotomies believe that they reduce the incidence of incontinence and damage to the perineum, that they protect the baby's head and that a cut is easier to repair than a tear. The current evidence does not support any of these claims.

How to avoid a tear or an episiotomy

One of the most common ways women try to avoid a tear or an episiotomy is to practise perineal massage. Recent research has shown that perineal massage can reduce overall the damage women experience to their perineums during birth. Other benefits of perineal massage include increasing the stretchiness of the tissue and helping to desensitise the area.

Perineal massage can be conducted by the pregnant women or her partner. It can be carried out using the following steps:

1 Wash hands.
2 Use a lubricant – either a water-based lubricant or a natural oil. Locate the perineum. This is the area between the vagina and anus. A mirror may be helpful for this step.
3 The woman usually finds it easier to use her thumbs to do perineal massage (partners can use index fingers). Insert thumbs into the vagina, then press downwards towards the anus and out towards the sides. This should be done until a burning sensation is experienced (not excessive). This pressure should be maintained until the area becomes a little numb, around two minutes.
4 Massage the area using a sweeping motion for a further three to four minutes, concentrating on scar tissue, if there is any.

Other methods used to avoid perineal damage include maintaining good nutrition during pregnancy (well-nourished tissue may be less likely to experience damage), and only pushing when you feel the urge during the second stage of labour, rather than being coached to push. This helps the second stage to be more gradual, therefore reducing the risk of perineal damage. A skilled midwife or doctor can guide a woman through the second stage to minimise tearing or the need for an episiotomy.

Lynn's first birth story

My waters broke with a pop three weeks before my due date. I had gone to bed for the night and was feeling very restless. As I rolled onto my side I heard the pop. Sitting upright for a minute, I felt a need to go to the toilet. In the bathroom I saw some light-pink blood and panicked. I was later told this was a show, caused by the mucus loosening from my cervix.

Not knowing what to do, I left my husband asleep while I went to wake up Mum and Dad. I then rang the hospital and was told to come straight in. I became fidgety and constantly checked my suitcase. I didn't want to go to the hospital anymore, as I now knew I had to, but Shane was wide awake and ready to go. Water was continually trickling down my legs and I kept needing heaps of pads.

Once at the hospital I was given an examination and was found to be 1.5 centimetres dilated, but not yet in labour. In fact, I didn't even know what labour was, as I had never even experienced a Braxton Hicks contraction. As I wasn't having contractions, I was put into a ward with two other women who had already had their babies. I was told that if nothing happened during the night, I would be induced in the morning.

At 8 am, after a sleepless night, I was moved to the induction room, where other women were sitting in lounge chairs waiting to be induced. Shane was now with me. My drip was set up and twenty minutes later the pains started. I gripped the arm of a nearby chair with every contraction until it passed. While timing one of my contractions, I heard a woman screaming in the distance. She must have been having a difficult time and it was really scaring me.

My contractions continued every twenty minutes, but were not unbearable. That is until midday, at which time they suddenly changed. Now coming every fifteen minutes, they had become a lot more painful.

At around 3 pm a woman and her husband came into the induction room and sat down. I said hi to her and she said hello back to me. She didn't even appear to be in labour. A short time later she got up and left. One hour later, while still sitting in the same chair, I saw this woman wheeled past in a wheelchair. She had already had her baby. I was still experiencing strong pains every ten to fifteen minutes, so was a little jealous, to say the least.

By 4 pm, with my drip still attached, I wanted to walk around. With each contraction I would lean against whatever I was next to, staying there until the pain subsided. Eventually, during one of my walks, I came across a bed in an empty room that looked inviting. At about the same time I was leaning against the bed, I had another contraction and started to cry. One of the midwives saw me and told me to go into the delivery room. Here she gave me an examination and put a fetal electrode onto our baby's head, to monitor our baby's condition. At about this time I felt the need for pain relief and asked the midwife for a gas mask. The gas took the edge off my pain, seeming to push it into the background, but I also felt pretty light-headed. I started to feel very uncomfortable and began tossing and turning between contractions, eventually finding myself more comfortable on my side with my legs up to my chest.

Soon I felt like passing a bowel motion, so the nurse put a pan underneath me. It was quickly removed, however, once they realised the baby's head was coming out. I was now given an injection of pethidine into my thigh, which didn't work. I then asked if I could have an epidural but was told, 'No, it's too late. You are having the baby now.' I was told they were giving me a birth cut to let the baby's head out. Still high on gas, I didn't care what they did.

After the episiotomy, I gave a few short pushes and out came our baby, slithering all the way. 'Is it a boy or a girl?' I asked straight away. 'Have a look,' came the reply. For some reason I was too scared and replied, 'Oh no,' so our baby was passed to Shane, who was holding him up in the air.

'It's a boy,' he said. I looked up and saw our baby's great big eyes looking around. I also noticed how gorgeous his hair looked. Pretty soon I was given an injection to help deliver the placenta. After I was sewn up, Shane went to the nursery with our baby. He watched him being cleaned and have his nose and throat cleared. Our baby was then weighed and measured.

Scott weighed 2863 grams and was 49 centimetres long – a good size for three weeks early, and being my first baby. He was born at 9.43 pm after thirteen hours of labour, seven hours of those pains being very strong. But it was a pain that I had coped with and considered worthwhile because of the wonderful son we now have.

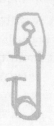

Nitrous oxide and oxygen (entonox)

Nitrous oxide and oxygen, or entonox, is also known as laughing gas. It is commonly used by dentists. The dosage varies from 30 per cent to 70 per cent nitrous oxide mixed with oxygen. The woman administers it herself by inhaling it through a face mask or mouthpiece during contractions. It takes around fifteen seconds to work, and if it is used from the very start of a contraction, it gives pain relief for most of the contraction. The woman continues to breathe on the mask or mouthpiece until the end of the contraction, then breathes air until the very beginning of the next contraction. The gas only works while it is being breathed in. It is effective for some women as it can act as a focal point, taking the edge off the contractions. However, some women find that the gas is not effective, and it may cause nausea and vomiting, drowsiness and confusion. There have been no obvious clinical long-term effects noted for mother or baby. However, little research has been done in this area.

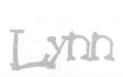

Lynn's second birth story

Some time between four and six in the evening I had a show, then at six o'clock on the dot I felt my first contraction. Ten minutes later, I had another one. I was 24 years old, 39 weeks pregnant and home by myself with our two-year-old son, Scott. Shane, my husband, was due at any time. 'I think I'll be having this baby tonight,' I told a very sceptical husband when he arrived home from work.

A knock on the door at 7 pm and we now had visitors, Vicky and Wesley, Shane's sister and brother-in-law. Feeling shy and not wanting them to see I was in labour, I tried to hide it from them and secretly pressed onto the table with every contraction I had. An hour later, I couldn't hide the pain any longer, so reluctantly I told Vicky and Wesley. To my utter amazement, Wesley became panicky and began timing my pains. His involvement made me embarrassed, and I was much happier once he left, but at least Shane now believed I was in labour. While our visitors were there, I rang the hospital and was told to come in when I felt like it.

Vicky and Wesley left at 9.30 pm, and at 10.15 pm Shane took our son over to Mum's place while I stayed behind. I tried to ease the pain by putting pressure onto my back. I had seen this done in a movie, where a woman pushed her back against the doorway every time she had a contraction. It didn't work for me. After that, I had a shower and got ready to leave for hospital.

We arrived at the hospital at about 11 pm. My contractions were now coming every five minutes and were very painful. The staff were so busy we had to wait an hour until another midwife started her shift before being seen. In the meantime, I lay on a bed I had spotted in one of the examination rooms. When a midwife finally did see me, she gave me an internal almost straight away. I was discovered to be 4 centimetres dilated – a very pleasant surprise.

Straight after the examination, we went to the delivery room. 'How long will it be before I give birth?' I asked the midwife. 'Well, my shift finishes at 8 am. You'll be having it before then,' she replied. I was happy with her light-hearted answer.

Shortly after the midwife left, I climbed off the bed to sit in a lounge chair. Still experiencing painful contractions every five minutes, I made myself as comfortable as I could, but it all became too much for me and I needed gas to take the edge off the pain. Breathing in gas whenever I needed it, I was immediately put into a different mood. Everything was in the background and was slightly unreal – including my painful contractions. It occurred to me that I should be careful what I said, as I had taken gas with the birth of our previous son and had said silly things.

An hour or so later, feeling rather restless and not knowing what I wanted, I decided to get off the chair. I lay on the examination bed, but soon realised I had made a mistake. It had been more comfortable on the chair. Thinking of the pain I was in for, I started to cry. A midwife approached me trying to discover what was wrong, but I was crying so much she couldn't understand me. Finally, I blurted it out: 'I'm scared.'

'Oh, well,' she said pleasantly, 'you should be experienced by now, this being your second baby.' Then she produced a long thing, which reminded me of chopsticks wrapped in brown paper. 'I'm just going to break your waters,' she said.

'Will it hurt?' I asked.

'Oh, you won't even feel it,' she replied in a convincing manner.

True, I didn't feel a thing, not even the water coming out. Once my waters were broken, I stayed on the bed for another hour or so, breathing in the gas when I needed it. Shane kept me company, but I hadn't seen much of the staff lately.

Despite Shane's presence, I was feeling very much alone. Looking back on it, I'm certain the gas was partly responsible for my unusual feelings. Later, when someone spoke to me, I heard it as an echo. 'Don't, don't, don't, don't, use, use, use, use, too, too, too, too, much, much, much, much, gas, gas, gas.' And I heard my own reply as, 'Okay, okay, okay.' I wasn't sure if I had said okay three times, or just once.

Lots of staff now arrived, including doctors and other assistants. At about the same time, things really started to happen. I was told to start pushing, but found I had no energy to do so. Because of this, it took me a long time to push our baby out – that is, compared to the three short pushes I had given to deliver our first son. Then I felt that familiar burning sensation and knew I was about to give birth. With one long final push, our baby's head came out, the rest of his body slithering out like jelly. It was a wonderful sensation.

Straight away, our baby was put onto my stomach, and I could see he was a boy. He was taken away to be cleaned, weighed and measured. I received a slight tear, but fortunately I only needed a few stitches. Once stitched, I promptly walked the few steps to the shower and had a wash. In the meantime, Shane was in the nursery with our baby.

Luke was born at 3 am. His birth weight was 3402 grams and his length 51 centimetres. I came home from the hospital the next day at about 4 pm feeling great. My first visitor, Auntie Margaret, couldn't believe it when she found me vacuuming and doing the housework.

Over the next week, a midwife from the hospital came and saw us every day, just to make sure we were all right, which was lovely.

Pethidine

Pethidine is a synthetic morphine-like drug given by injection, normally into the thigh or buttock, to help women in labour relax and cope with the pain. It acts on nerve cells in the spine and brain and is thought to inhibit pain messages reaching the brain, therefore reducing the amount of pain experienced. It takes around fifteen to twenty minutes to work and lasts for two to three hours.

One of the major problems in using pethidine is that it doesn't work for all women. In one study, nearly half the women said it provided no pain relief at all, while the others said it provided excellent pain relief. Pethidine can help the cervix to dilate more quickly in some women by helping them to relax. On the down side, however, it is known to have a number of side effects, which include sedation, confusion, disorientation, nausea, vomiting, difficulty in coping with contractions, hallucinations, respiratory depression, low blood pressure and allergic reaction. For the baby, pethidine has no advantages. It passes across the placenta and can cause breathing difficulties after the birth (particularly if pethidine is given to the baby's mother one to three hours before the birth). Babies are more likely to be jaundiced and experience breastfeeding difficulties for a number of days.

Cathy's birth story

I had a good pregnancy that had been fairly uneventful, but, because I live in a small country town where the hospital is not equipped to handle an emergency, I had to travel two and a half hours to a larger hospital for check-ups and to give birth.

At 41 weeks, I began feeling frustrated and tired of waiting for the baby. Thinking I was experiencing contractions, I admitted myself to hospital where I stayed overnight, but I was sent home the next morning when it turned out to be a false alarm. I was staying at my grandparents' place and I continued waiting impatiently for something to happen.

Three days later, at about 1 am, I felt my contractions were starting again, so I rang the hospital and was told to come in. A fetal monitor was attached to my stomach, but once again it showed no contractions. Feeling extremely disappointed, I was very glad when they asked me to stay, planning to induce me in two days time. The night before the planned induction I was given some sleeping tablets. Fifteen minutes later, at 9.15 pm, I felt three pops in my stomach and my waters went everywhere. A midwife took me to the birthing suite where she did an examination. The examination hurt a lot and I was only 2 centimetres dilated. I was now given the option to stay where I was or to go back to my room. I decided to go back to my room, but first made a phone call to my partner, Peter.

It was 9.30 pm and my contractions were five minutes apart, with pain in my lower back. They were quite different from anything I had heard or read about. One would hit me like a wave, slowly getting stronger until it would peak, then start going away. Five minutes later I would feel another contraction, only the second would not be like the first. Instead of building up to one peak of very strong pain, it would build up to two peaks. My third contraction would be the same as the first, and the fourth like the second, and so on. My unusual contractions surprised me, as did the fact that I had no build-up to this strong labour, just immediate, full-on pains.

Peter arrived at about 9.45 pm, and from then stayed by my side. He was doing his best to comfort me but was unable to actually help. No position seemed to ease the pain. I tried standing, leaning over, rocking my hips and sitting down, but every time I had a contraction my knees would buckle and I could hardly stand. So getting into the shower wasn't an option either, although some time later I did get into the shower. My knees were still giving way with every contraction, so I couldn't stay in there for very long. The midwife was really good and asked if I was all right, telling me I must let her know if I wanted anything.

Soon afterwards I did become a bit distressed, so I tried the gas, but I only had one suck before deciding to stop. It was making me feel weird and I hated not being in control of myself. What felt like hours later, I ended up taking pethidine, but this didn't help one little bit. It just made me tired, putting me to sleep between contractions. This meant that I was unable to anticipate and prepare for my contractions, so was jumping from pain out of my sleep with every one I had.

Peter was looking a bit harassed. He was not sure what to do. I began to feel upset that I had taken the pethidine because it was going to affect the baby as well. No longer coping terribly well with the contractions, I asked for an epidural. Half an hour later, at 6 am, I was finally given pain relief when the epidural took hold. A monitor was also attached to record my contractions. The midwives now discovered I was only 3 centimetres dilated. Also, my contractions had stopped (probably because of the epidural), so I was given a drip to restart them.

I was no longer in pain, so Peter went back to our room and had a sleep, and I began sleeping between examinations. Every ten minutes my blood pressure was being checked to make sure it wasn't dropping. By now, I had a different midwife, as the midwives had changed shifts, but I was never left alone. Two student nurses were also with me.

By 9 am the midwife could see my baby's head. I asked someone if they could wake up Peter, as I wanted him present for the birth. The midwife went to ring the doctor to ask if she could stop the epidural, but the doctor said there was no reason to do this. I was very glad about his reply, as I didn't want the pain to return. The doctor arrived wearing a medical gown and gloves. The anaesthetist arrived as well. Now I had the doctor, anaesthetist, two student nurses, the midwife and Peter present. I wasn't the least worried by my large audience, as by now I couldn't have cared less, nor was I frightened by my impending delivery.

As I couldn't feel the lower half of my body, the anaesthetist told me he was going to let me know when a contraction came, so I could breathe deeply and begin pushing. I did push when told to, but I wasn't able to make anything happen. Another midwife arrived with a variety of suction caps and the doctor chose one to pull our baby out. Now I became really upset. My nephew had been delivered using suction and his head had become very bruised, staying that way for three months.

Still flat on my back, I watched the doctor pull our baby from within me, but didn't feel a thing. The baby started crying and was placed onto my stomach straight away. I was crying and the baby was screaming in my ear. I didn't know what sex it was.

Not long afterwards, the midwife took our baby to be weighed, checked and measured. I heard the midwife ask Peter whether it was a boy or a girl. 'I don't know,' he replied.

'It's a girl!' she happily told us.

Throughout my whole pregnancy I had felt I was having a girl. I heard the doctor say he could hear a click in her hip, but it turned out that she didn't have any problems.

They wrapped our daughter and gave her to Peter, who was over-whelmed and crying with joy. We were both crying with happiness, but I was also crying from distress, as I was a little worried about what the suction cap might have done.

While our baby was being bathed, I was stitched (I tore, but didn't feel a thing as the epidural was still making me numb). I then asked if I could go. I felt so good I thought I could just get up and walk away! However, the midwife replied, 'Oh no, dear. I don't think you could do that.' She then explained that I would be unable to walk because of the epidural still numbing me from my waist down.

Soon my baby was brought to me to be fed. She was 3750 grams, 55 centimetres long and just beautiful. Her Apgar scores were 10 and 10. There was nothing wrong with her hips and she had no bruising on her head. All of which made me extremely happy.

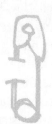

The pros and cons of pain relief

Many women having their first baby are unaware that the choices they make during labour can actually make their pains stronger or, alternatively, more bearable. The need for drugs is less likely if you are coping with the pain and feel in control of what is happening. Giving birth in a birth centre is one way to maintain control. Having your own support people also helps.

During labour, your cervix, which was previously closed, opens in preparation for the birth of your child. For your cervix to open, your body produces hormones that stimulate contractions, often felt as tightenings across your stomach or back. These tightenings are felt by different women in different ways and in varying degrees of strength. For many women, the pain is very strong and extremely unpleasant, especially during later first-stage labour (transition). Pain relief is often offered to women at this time.

Pain relief can sometimes be a little misleading, as in some cases the relief gained from drugs may be minimal. Drugs may not produce the desired effect and may increase the sense of pain. Pethedine, for example, can sometimes take the edge off your pain, but it can also make you sleepy and therefore unprepared for the next contraction, thus interfering with your ability to cope. If given late in labour, pethidine can also make both mother and baby very sleepy after the birth. Instead of enjoying those first exciting moments, you may find yourself falling asleep or unable to comprehend what has happened. A drowsy baby may initally have problems with breastfeeding. Mothers who have taken pethidine are more likely to have infants with lower Apgar scores.

Some pain relief is difficult to synchronise. If nitrous oxide (or gas) is taken too close to the peak of your contraction, it has no time to take effect. Of course, the use of an epidural or a nitrous oxide mask can give great relief to a mother experiencing a long and painful labour. So, the use of drugs should not be discarded – just put into its rightful place. Used when medically necessary or when the pain is more than a woman can take, pain-relieving drugs can greatly assist a labour.

Jenny's birth story

Grahame took me to the hospital at 8.30 pm. The midwife put some prostaglandin gel in my vagina and told me nothing much would happen for the first few hours. Fortunately she gave me a couple of sleeping tablets, otherwise I would never have been able to sleep. Grahame left to go home, with instructions to phone the hospital in the morning if he hadn't heard from us by then.

I awoke at midnight with mild contractions almost exactly three minutes apart. These continued until I fell asleep at about 3 am, only to be awoken two hours later with contractions still coming every three minutes. When the doctor arrived at 8.30 am, nothing had changed. The doctor believed I was still only 2 centimetres dilated and suggested another dose of the gel to see if it would speed things along.

During the morning, my contractions came closer together and became slightly stronger. I kept on my feet as much as possible, pacing up and down the hospital corridors. At around 11 am, the midwife suggested a spa – so we moved to the delivery suite. I almost started crying when I realised I would give birth in the exact same room where I had delivered my last baby. I remembered all the emotions surging through me immediately following Jamie's delivery.

The warm water was a great relief for my back and legs, as I'd now been on my feet for a few hours. I spent one and a half hours in the spa, but when I got out my contractions had almost stopped.

At 1.30 pm I was still only 2 to 3 centimetres dilated. The head had come down only a little further and was not yet properly engaged. The next course of action was to rupture my membranes in the hope that things would speed up a little. The contractions did come a little closer, every five to six minutes, and intensified quite drastically. The pain would suddenly peak from nowhere, leaving me reeling and unable to breathe, and lasting one and a half minutes.

After a while I began to worry that I might start hyperventilating. I lay on the bed and, at one point, felt very sick because I had once again made the mistake of trying the gas. I should have known better. Two breaths and I promptly threw up. This was when I started thinking of other forms of pain relief, especially since I still had a long way to go. I quickly dismissed pethidine, as I was unsure of what it would do. I tentatively asked the midwife if I could have an epidural. The anaesthetist was called and by 4.30 pm all the pain had vanished. What bliss.

The most frightening thing was having to lie absolutely still while this was done. My greatest fear was having a contraction and involuntarily moving in spite of my husband and the midwife holding me down. Anyway, all went well and a pleasant numbness set in. Although I could still tell when a contraction came, there was no pain associated with it. The oddest thing was my body getting the shakes from the epidural, although this settled after a while.

My body was now wired for sound. Not only did I have a drip in my arm for fluids, but around my tummy I had a monitor to measure my contractions and the baby's heart rate. (Retrospectively, a very reassuring sound.) They say that one dose of the epidural can last between two and four hours, but after only one and a half hours I started to feel the contractions again and asked for a top-up. It took ten to fifteen minutes for the midwife to obtain the anaesthetist's okay, so I'm glad I asked for it when I did, as the contractions soon became very painful again. She gave me the top-up at 6.30 pm, and this one numbed me for longer.

As time went on, I started to feel pushes against my pelvis. The doctor examined me just before 8.30 pm, and I was still only 4 to 5 centimetres dilated, with contractions still five minutes apart. The epidural had been a good choice – the doctor indicated his approval. By 8.30 pm I was given an Syntocinon drip to bring on stronger contractions. This did it almost immediately. I was glad I'd been given a second top-up, as I was gradually beginning to feel pain in my pelvis from the baby pushing against it.

At 9.30 pm there was a change in shifts. One midwife going off duty said I should prepare myself in case the doctor decided to do a caesarean, as the baby's heartbeat was dropping every time I had a contraction. She also told me the baby's head was facing sideways, not down, and unless it turned it would not fit through my pelvis. The thought I had then was that, knowing my luck, the baby would have a large head (which turned out to be true) and might not easily fit through anyway.

The new midwife (like the previous one) was very supportive and, as I was the only one they had in labour that evening, stayed with me while she sent Grahame to have a cup of tea. She told me our doctor was on his way. Then I started to feel a huge urge to push. The midwife said this was the best news she could hear, and told me to go ahead. I didn't feel so convinced. How could I be ready to push at 9.45 when at 8.30 I'd been only 5 centimetres dilated and at 9.30 the baby's head was still facing the wrong way – and why was the epidural no longer taking the pain away? I wasn't feeling the contractions, but the pain as the head came down was definitely there. I as good as refused to push, as I'd convinced myself I wasn't ready and would only swell up and hurt myself if the baby's head was facing the wrong way. I really wished someone would take a look. Then my husband, who had come back, also urged me to push.

At last another nurse came and examined me. And yes, the head was indeed starting to appear. It was only about one inch away. That was all the encouragement I needed. My husband held one leg and the midwife the other, and at last the doctor appeared. I was half on one side, but still on my back, and all of a sudden they could see the top of the head. The head slowly started to come out and I reached down and touched it. (I had promised myself I would do so while pregnant.) I suddenly felt that I wasn't getting any further and the doctor suggested a small cut. (He couldn't do it fast enough!) He told me to pant, which I gladly did, as I had just finished a contraction.

The head came out almost instantly, followed by the rest of the body at 10.06 pm. Our baby was lifted onto my lower abdomen, as the cord was very short (as with my first delivery). She was a little purple and covered in vernix, but she was the most beautiful baby girl I'd ever seen. She had black hair, dark eyes, long fingers and was definitely not wrinkly. Both my husband and I were surprised it was a girl. Our baby's Apgar scores were 8 and 9. She weighed 3470 grams and was 57 centimetres long. She had a big head, with a circumference of 36.5 centimetres.

After the birth, I started to shake uncontrollably, probably from the epidural, and it took a while for me to calm down. Our baby's neck was very strong, right from the beginning. As she lay in her crib while they cleaned me and sat me up, I saw her turn her head around and lift it up. She was trying to see behind her. I put her to my breast and she managed to suckle well. Later I was taken to my room. My legs felt like lead from the epidural, but I still had strength in them.

At around midnight, my husband finally got a chance to head home, and I tried to get some sleep. Catherine let me sleep until 6 am, which I was very grateful for. She was a little jaundiced in the beginning, but that gradually faded. I remember having worried that I could ever find love for another child, especially when I loved my son so much. But, looking at Catherine, it now seemed silly to have worried about this, as I couldn't imagine not having love for both my children.

Caesarean deliveries

A caesarean birth is a major surgical operation performed to remove the baby from its mother's uterus by cutting through the walls of the abdomen and womb. A caesarean birth can be carried out using an epidural anaesthetic (the mother is awake) or using a general anaesthetic (the mother is asleep). It may be a planned or elective caesarean that is performed before labour begins, or an emergency procedure after labour has commenced. There are a number of other reasons why a caesarean birth may be recommended. These include:

- the mother has severe pre-eclampsia
- the mother has pelvic disproportion
- the labour fails to progress
- the baby is in distress
- the baby is in a position that makes it unable to be born vaginally
- the placenta is in the wrong position (placenta praevia)
- there are concerns for the health of the mother and/or baby.

There are risks associated with caesarean birth, such as infection, bleeding, problems with the anaesthetic, problems with women's fertility after the birth, and increased risk of problems with the placenta for future births, and babies may have a higher incidence of respiratory distress syndrome compared to those who have undergone the process of labour.

There is no doubt that caesarean sections are life-saving procedures. However, it is known that in Western countries the caesarean birth rate is high. Caesarean births sometimes occur for less clear-cut reasons. For example:

- previous caesarean birth (most women can give birth vaginally after a caesarean birth)
- it is the woman's first baby and she is an older mother
- the mother has a history of infertility
- twins
- breech birth.

Fiona's first birth story – caesarean by general anaesthetic

My doctor considered me a neurotic mother by the time I made my third demand for an ultrasound in a fifteen-week period. 'Mother feels the fetus is dead,' read the note attached to my request. I didn't see that note until I had opened it ready to give to the ultrasound people, and they all cracked up with laughter. But my concern stemmed from a miscarriage I had suffered several months earlier.

Apart from this particular incident, my pregnancy was a lot of fun. I laughed all the way through it, staying up late with friends, playing cards until 3 am and eating whatever I liked – especially liquorice and milk mixed together. It was a wonderful pregnancy that I really enjoyed.

Then, before I knew it, I was two weeks overdue. Impatient and feeling very irritable, I was with my husband, Joe, at his cousin and my friend Mary's place when jokingly everyone said I was in labour and should go to the hospital. I said the time wasn't right. Joe and I went straight home to bed. At 3.45 am, however, I realised I was having regular contractions every fifteen minutes. At first I just lay there enjoying them, as these pains were my first experience of labour and were only mild. Then, just after 9 am, I woke Joe. He quickly got dressed, grabbed my bag and we headed off for the hospital.

At the hospital, my first examination found me only 1 centimetre dilated. We live so close to the hospital, we were told to go home and relax for a few hours. Setting back for home, we felt disappointed and let down. However, within minutes of arriving home, I went into the full throes of labour. Arriving back at the hospital, we were met by an orderly waiting with a wheelchair to take me to the maternity ward. The midwives checked me a second time to discover I was still only 1 centimetre dilated. I couldn't believe it.

'I've got to be at least 5 centimetres,' I said to the nurse. 'No,' she said. 'Go grab yourself a tank of gas, then hit the showers.'

I did exactly as she suggested, standing in the shower and sucking on the gas. I had hot water pouring down my back, which was really soothing, and gas, which was bringing a smile to my face. After becoming as wrinkled as a prune from head to toe, I decided to go into the maternity lounge and make use of their beanbag and other facilities. I wanted as natural a birth as possible, wanting to feel the contractions. I restricted myself to gas only while coping with the pain.

After three hours in this room, Joe felt he needed a break. I was coping well, so Joe phoned Mary, who turned up ten minutes later. Mary was really supportive, rubbing my back, chatting and keeping me company. It was very comforting to have a female friend present. Joe returned, and not long afterwards my pains became really severe and I began to feel like pushing. The midwife asked me to come into one of the delivery rooms. The next thing I recall is that I had a baby monitor attached and was *really* feeling the pains. The gas was no longer enough for me. (I later attributed this extra pain to being placed on my back.) Whenever the monitor was removed, I rolled from my back onto my side, which did help slightly. The pain was getting so severe that after a while Joe couldn't stand watching me.

Still in a lot of pain, I kept asking the midwife when the doctor would be coming.

'Six pm,' I was finally told. When he did arrive, I wished that he hadn't. He walked in like a man with a mission and without a word grabbed an instrument that looked like a crochet hook and proceeded to break my waters. After the fifth or sixth attempt (and ear-piercing screams from me), he gave up. I told him his reputation for being gentle had just been shattered.

Then the doctor told me, 'You're only 2 centimetres dilated. And that's being generous. You will need a Syntocinon drip to speed things up.' At that point, my idea of a natural labour went out the window.

Now I was on a drip, the pain was incredibly severe. A nurse came in to check on me and soon realised it had been turned up too high. The contractions were coming every couple of minutes and were absolutely unbearable. Then, in the middle of all the pain, something funny happened. Only days earlier, I'd heard that a baby's heartbeat doesn't register on the monitor while the mother is experiencing a contraction. I had even noticed this myself. It wasn't until one of my more severe contractions that Mary (my backbone) suddenly thought the baby was dead or something was dreadfully wrong. Without saying a word she simply ran out of the room screaming for a doctor. I sat upright and started yelling, 'Mary, Mary, it's all right.' But it was too late. A barrage of nurses and midwives came charging in, and I was the one who had to comfort them (especially Mary).

The doctor had previously told me the drip would be out by 10.30 pm, but by this time I was screaming for every drug in the house. The contractions were coming thick and fast, and I couldn't bear it any more. To make matters worse, I suddenly noticed that the baby's heart rate had gone up. *I* was now the one worried about the baby.

Finally a midwife came in. She gave me some pethidine through the drip, which didn't help. I felt totally drugged, but still in pain. Then, eventually, the doctor arrived. With very little comment he told me the baby was in distress and this had gone on for too long. 'Sorry, Fiona,' he said, 'but this will be an emergency caesarean.'

This is when I turned to Joe and asked, 'Is something wrong with the baby?'

With his lip quivering, Joe passionately replied, 'No, nothing is wrong.'

I believed Joe and relaxed a little, but if the doctor had been the one to tell me, I wouldn't have believed him, as I no longer had any faith in him.

In preparation for my caesarean, a **catheter** was inserted. The next thing I remember, three women were standing at the end of my bed, one of them saying, 'What is this?' Apparently my waters had broken at the same time my catheter was inserted, even though this area was not related to the other.

Soon someone was saying, 'Relax, Fiona, we're just putting you under. It will all be over very soon.'

It wasn't until the moment I realised I couldn't breathe that I also realised I was still on the operating table and could hear voices (even though I was under the anaesthetic). I couldn't talk nor move to let them know I had woken up. Trying to think rationally, I realised this tube must be doing the breathing for me, but I still had to let someone know I was awake. Although my senses were working, I felt no pain, but I was panicking because I couldn't breathe naturally. Concentrating as hard as I could, I put all my fear and efforts into moving my leg. When it finally did move, I kicked the doctor.

'This woman is still awake,' he said with great surprise. 'Fiona, calm down,' he kept saying.

By now, I could also move one of my hands, so pointed to my mouth, gargling to the anaesthetist next to me, 'I can't breathe.'

'Sorry, Mrs. Sorry, Mrs. Sorry, Mrs,' was all he could say.

'Quick, put her under,' the doctor now said.

The next thing I remember, I was in recovery feeling pretty sore and sorry. I had almost forgotten I was having a baby. I saw my husband, Joe, who said, 'He's got my beak,' pointing to his nose. After hearing that, I must have dozed off, although I'm not sure for how long. When I awoke, a nurse was saying, 'Would you like to see your son?'

'Yes,' I replied. So she brought him in to me. Rolling over to my side, I looked at my little son and, with every ounce of affection, said, 'You little rat,' after which I promptly went back to sleep. When they had taken me into the delivery room, Joe had followed hot on the heels of the doctors and nurses, and managed to see our baby minutes after he was born.

The nurses rushed our baby straight to the emergency nursery, but before they could get him there, Joe made them put Zac down for a minute so he could take a photograph. Joe knew how much I had wanted to be awake for the birth and knew this photograph would be very precious to me. After that, they rushed poor Zac off to have his stomach pumped because of the meconium he had swallowed.

Zac's weight at birth was 3350 grams and he was 53 centimetres long.

Dianne's first birth story

Dianne had developed pre-eclampsia and was to be induced. Her story continues from Part 1.

It was seventeen days before my due date. Thursday morning had come and the induction was about to be set up. Brett was now with me. Lying flat on my back, I was given drugs to start my contractions, our baby being monitored at the same time. But nothing happened. They kept putting the dosage up, but basically nothing was happening. Because of my high blood pressure, I had to stay on my back, so I just lay there, watching the monitor going up and down.

Hours passed and still nothing was happening (except my blood pressure was staying up). I was now getting frustrated and bored. When a caesarean was finally suggested at 2 pm, Brett said, 'Hooray. Things are finally going to happen.' But my heart sank. Although I had known of the possibility of a caesarean, I had never actually expected it to eventuate. 'If I have to have a caesarean, please can I have an epidural rather than a general anaesthetic?' I asked the doctor. 'Yes, of course,' came his reply.

An interesting change of heart now came from my husband, who hadn't even wanted to be present for the birth. Suddenly he wanted to be present for the impending caesarean. This change in attitude floored me.

The anaesthetist came in and the epidural was set up. It took well. I was numb from my waist down. I was now ready for the caesarean when the doctor came in, but instead of saying, 'Let's go,' he informed me two emergency caesareans had come in and they weren't able to deliver our baby until they had finished with these. So here I was on hold.

Nearly two hours passed, during which time my epidural was kept topped up, but because of the long delay I began to get the epidural shakes. My teeth were chattering and I was shivering and shaking uncontrollably. (Apparently this normally happens a couple of hours after the baby has been born.) It was now 4 pm and the doctors were finally ready for me. They wheeled me into the operating room. An anaesthetist sat up near my head, poking around with various tubes, then got up and left. A few minutes later he came back and sat next to me. Leaning right over me, he said, 'It's me, darling. I'm here.' It was Brett, dressed up in a green uniform, mask and hat. Still shaking and chattering, I thought I would fall off the bed. I looked up at the reflection of the operating lights to see them painting my stomach, and it suddenly occurred to me that a caesarean was not just a way of delivery, it was major surgery for me. This thought upset me a lot.

They put this big screen across my stomach so I couldn't see anything, but, just as they started operating, I noticed that Brett was peering over the screen to see what was going on. Normally he wouldn't have even watched an operation on television! What happened next surprised me.

'Well, come on, give us a push. Push your baby out,' I was told.

As I was numb from my waist down, I didn't know if I was pushing or not, so gave this grunt and hoped that I was. Then the doctor brought out forceps and began to pull out our baby. The next thing I remember is that the clock on the wall read 4.25 pm, and I remember thinking, 'The baby will be born at about 4.30.' Then, all of a sudden, they whipped her out at 4.25 pm. They carried her up somewhere behind my head, but stopped to show her to me. She was then taken to be weighed and measured. Our baby came back all clean and wrapped, and was given to Brett for a cuddle. She weighed 3195 grams and was 50.5 centimetres long.

The doctor was sewing me up. I was shaking and shivering so much I couldn't work out how he could do it. After he had finished, I was taken to the recovery room, while Brett went up to the nursery to be with our baby. She was in shock from having been born so quickly, and had lost heat, so she had to stay in a crib with an electric blanket until her temperature stabilised.

In the meantime, different midwives kept coming up to me, telling me what a beautiful little girl I had. 'Congratulations,' they kept saying, 'You have a beautiful daughter.' But I couldn't understand what all the fuss was about. I was still in mild shock and half out of it, having just been through unexpected major surgery.

Fiona's second birth story

Fiona

My second pregnancy was much more difficult than my first. My sciatic nerve kept twinging, and the pain was incredible. I'd yell out loud, then have to sit down, attracting a lot of attention to myself. Once, at five months, I had to calm down my mother-in-law, who thought I was letting out a labour yell. It took a lot of explaining before I had convinced her that it was my age – I was 36 – and that my body wasn't handling the pregnancy particularly well this time around. Morning sickness was also a problem and I felt constantly lethargic.

With an uncomfortable pregnancy almost over, I was looking forward to a natural birth. I had been told by all the staff at the clinic that there should be no need for a second caesarean. However, at 38 weeks, the head obstetrician said, 'Forget it. Don't put your body through the same thing,' meaning my previous 24-hour labour followed by an emergency caesarean. She booked me in for a caesarean the following week. I was admitted the night before my caesarean. I had the best night's sleep ever since Zac's birth two years ago, as he was still waking every three hours. So a night on my own was wonderful.

Joe arrived early the next morning, happily anticipating the birth and happy in the knowledge that he wouldn't be going through the dreadful worry of my first labour. At 9 am an orderly told us it was time to go upstairs. Joe was told the epidural would only take fifteen minutes and to wait in the adjacent room. I was taken into the preparation room and two doctors explained what was going to happen, telling me it was a simple procedure. I remember dreading the thought of a needle going into my spine, but the local anaesthetic was nothing more than a pinprick.

Two doctors were present – one older and one younger. The older doctor explained the procedure to the younger one, while pointing out places on my back. Once he had finished talking, he promptly left, leaving me with the young doctor, an elderly nurse and a male nurse. Everything was fine until the doctor made an incision into my back for the tube to be placed. He seemed to be having problems placing it along my spinal cord. At this stage I was experiencing a terrible pain at the top of my right leg. Bending over in a fetal position is very uncomfortable when you are nine months pregnant, and being told not to move made things even worse. So at this stage I needed to hold someone's hand. The elderly nurse volunteered, but then wished she hadn't. With every movement the doctor made, the pain caused me to squeeze the poor woman's hand with such force that I thought her bones were going to break, and the wince on her face proved my prognosis to be close. Meanwhile, Joe was being prepped for theatre, being told to relax and that everything was fine.

Half an hour later, the doctor was still trying to insert the tube into the correct channel. By now, the oxygen mask I was wearing was filling up with tears, which were bubbling back in my face. The poor nurse whose hand I was pulverising also had tears in her eyes – both in sympathy for me and also from her own pain. The next thing I heard, the doctor told the nurse to quickly get the other doctor (who was sitting next to Joe reading his newspaper). Joe got up and began pacing around, as he knew the procedure was taking too long. When the nurse arrived to collect the doctor, she bustled Joe out of the room saying everything was fine, but Joe didn't believe her.

When the older doctor came back, the young doctor explained he had encountered blood rather than spinal fluid. Hearing this sent a cold shiver up my spine. The young doctor then said I might have to go under a general anaesthetic, but, because of my previous experience, this was the last thing I wanted. So I said quickly, 'No, please keep trying.'

So the experienced doctor took over, and after another twenty minutes finally got it through. With great relief, the nurse's hands were finally freed, and I lay down, waiting for the epidural to work. After a few minutes, they wheeled me into the delivery room, where moments later Joe joined me dressed in green. The doctor who had succeeded with the epidural put a block of ice onto my foot and moved it all the way up my leg, asking if I could feel anything cold. To my joy, I was numb from the waist down.

Next followed a lot of hustle and bustle. A green partition was put in front of me and Joe was given a stool to sit on. Nurses ran around madly clanging instruments, which rang in my ears. Then a very jolly male face peeped over the partition saying he was going to put in a catheter. I asked him if it would hurt, as my previous one had, but he said because of my epidural I wouldn't feel a thing. Then before I knew it he was finished.

Next a doctor came in and introduced herself, telling me she would be delivering the baby. I found this rather surprising, as she was not my doctor. She explained there would be lots of pulling and tugging, and if I felt nauseous to let her know so they could give me something to stop it. And I replied, 'Let the games begin.'

Joe stayed huddled close to my head, only venturing away to look once or twice over the partition. At one stage during the operation, the tugging was so amazing that my whole body was being jolted backwards and forwards like someone trying to shake me awake. I even asked what was happening, but the reply was, 'It's normal, it's normal.' Half an hour later, Alex was out, the first comment being, 'What a dog.' This was because of his almost shoulder-length black hair, but I could not see him, so immediately took offence.

Joe stood up and went to him. I saw Alex for a split second over the partition before the nurse and Joe quickly took him across the room to an awaiting crib. He was then wrapped and brought over to me so that I could see him. He did look a little like a long-haired German shepherd. All I could see was hair! He was only 43 centimetres long, but weighed 3896 grams, and was built like a sumo wrestler. I found him absolutely beautiful.

Then Joe and the nurse left with our baby to clean him up while I was left with the doctor to be stitched up. I was now on my own. That is until I looked up to see this very bruised hand on my shoulder. It was the same nurse I had tortured earlier, asking me how I felt. 'Fine,' I replied, 'But how is your hand?'

After it was all finished, I was taken to the recovery room and this beautiful little sumo was placed in my arms. My husband and I had thought of many names, Alex being one of them, so when we discovered the name tag on the nurse with the bruised hand was Alex, this made it final for us. We now have two healthy boys, Alex and Zac, born two years and two days apart, and they are both absolutely gorgeous!

Placenta praevia

The placenta is usually in the upper part of the uterus. However, in some cases it attaches in the lower part of the uterus, and is known as placenta praevia. Placenta praevia occurs in 0.5 per cent of all pregnancies. There are different degrees of placenta praevia. Grade 1 is where most of the placenta is in the upper section of the uterus. Grade 2 is where part of the placenta is located in the lower segment of the uterus and the edge of the placenta reaches the opening of the uterus (cervix). Grade 3 is where part of the placenta is covering the internal opening of the cervix. Grade 4 is the most severe form of placenta praevia, where the placenta is located directly over the top of the cervical opening. The main problem of placenta praevia during pregnancy is the risk of bleeding. This needs careful monitoring and sometimes requires hospitalisation. With Grades 1 and 2 a vaginal birth is possible. With Grades 3 and 4 the only option is a caesarean birth, as the placenta covers the opening through which the baby has to pass.

Trial of labour

This is where a vaginal birth is attempted even though there are some factors present that may mean that a caesarean birth is more likely. These factors include having had a previous caesarean, where the placenta is low or if the baby appears to be very large. If the labour progresses normally, the woman will end up giving birth vaginally.

All births large and small

In some respects, babies are a law unto themselves. When it comes time to be born they do not always take the easy way out. Some babies come early, some present with their face, others with their bottoms, and multiple births require careful attention. However, as these stories show, most babies are resilient and sooner or later make their way into the world.

Face presentation

A **face presentation** occurs when the baby extends its head backwards so that its face is presenting at the cervix. Although it is quite rare, occurring only in around 1 in 500 births, it is more common when a woman has had one or more babies because the tone of her stomach is more lax and does not hold the baby in position. Other reasons for face presentation include the pelvis being an unusual shape, there being too much amniotic fluid surrounding the baby, or if there is an abnormality with the baby's head or neck. A normal birth is possible, though the labour is often prolonged. When the baby is born, they often have marked swelling and bruising to the face.

Wendy's birth story

Wendy's baby was in face presentation and the head had not engaged. Her story continues from Part 1.

When I was ten days overdue, my independent midwife discovered the baby's head to be getting lower, but it was still not engaged, so we discussed having ultrasounds done in a few days' time. This was also the day the builder finished extensions on our house, so Richard and I immediately began our big clean-up. We moved furniture into our newly built room. Then, when everything was done, we sat down and had our dinner. Straight after dinner I felt it – my first contraction.

'Oh no,' was my immediate thought. 'I'm tired already, but here I am starting labour, and all I need is a good night's sleep.'

I was booked to have the baby at the birth centre. My midwife was to be contacted so she could attend the birth once I was in labour. I had to travel by boat and then by car to get to the centre. Throughout my pregnancy, lots of people had kept telling me to travel into the city before I came into labour, but my midwife and I had always thought I'd have plenty of time once my labour started. Now my contractions were coming every five minutes and quickly getting stronger, so we immediately got into the boat, travelling for twenty minutes across the water, followed by the half-hour car trip to my mother's. Here we spent the night. (There was no rush after all.) I was sitting in the chair dozing off between contractions, while Richard spent the night sleeping on the floor next to me.

At about 6 am I decided I wanted to go to the birth centre. My midwife met us there. Looking back, it was probably too soon to go, as I was only 2 centimetres dilated.

Almost immediately after arriving at the birth centre we could hear a woman in the late first stage of her labour. She was in the spa sucking on the gas mask, moaning and groaning and sounding very distressed. She sounded so lonely that I started to cry, and said to my mum, 'I don't want to get to that stage that she is at.'

For the next few hours I spent my time sitting down or walking around, trying out as many positions as I could to make myself comfortable. At about lunchtime, a girlfriend turned up with some food. It was a very nice thought, but I couldn't eat a thing.

Every half hour my midwife checked the baby's heartbeat to make sure it was all right, but didn't pressure me at all when it came to being examined. She totally left it up to me to ask when I wanted this. After 24 hours of contractions, I did ask my midwife to examine me, but was still only 3 centimetres dilated. I now knew it wasn't going to work and I had a strong feeling something was wrong.

My midwife thought the baby was probably stuck in a face presentation. She said I could keep going for another hour if I wanted to, to see how it went. But I said, 'No, I don't think it's going to make any difference.' I felt it was time to move on, and I needed a rest from those contractions.

My midwife was happy to have me admitted to the labour ward. I was taken across to have a Syntocinon drip inserted and an epidural to cope with that. Once admitted to the labour ward, my own midwife could no longer have any say in what happened. Regardless of this, however, she came with me, never leaving my side.

After four hours on the drip, a young registrar examined me. 'You are fully dilated,' he said. 'You can start pushing whenever you feel like it.' So we waited for the epidural to wear off, which took about half an hour, then everyone began encouraging me to push through the contractions, even though I didn't feel like it. In fact, it really hurt me to push – it felt like a knife was being pushed into my bottom. Regardless of this, I pushed really hard for about two hours (so hard I gave myself haemorrhoids). I remember thinking, something must be wrong; I am a very fit person, yet people who aren't fit can push their babies out.

After three hours of this, I said, 'Please, we've got to get help.' So we moved into the next level of intervention.

Pretty soon, a different doctor came to examine me, saying, 'What are you pushing for? The baby is presenting face first – you shouldn't be pushing at all.'

He now discussed what was going to happen. He said the ventouse suction wouldn't work and that he would try forceps, but he felt this wouldn't work either. He said he wanted me to go to theatre to be prepped for a caesarean section, but once there he was first going to try to turn the baby with forceps.

I said, 'Fine, go ahead.' At this point I no longer felt I could cope with even one more contraction. I was self-administering epidural top-ups and was now told to continue doing this whenever I needed it.

Pretty soon a kind of three-ringed circus was wheeled in. I was surrounded by people asking questions or collecting blood samples. I remember one young registrar about to take blood from my arm saying to me, 'This is going to hurt.' I just laughed at him. I had experienced such a lot of pain already that having my arm pricked was absolutely nothing compared to that.

There was also an anaesthetist asking me medical history questions. In the middle of one of her questions, I had a huge contraction and stopped talking. 'What's wrong, dear?' she asked. 'She's in labour,' three people replied at once.

I don't know whether it was the top-up of the epidural, or something else, but my head began to spin badly. I had an overwhelming feeling that if I closed my eyes I would die. I honestly believed I was looking at the last things in my life.

Feeling like I was going to have a fit, I told them, 'I think I am going to die.' I now saw everyone begin to panic and remember seeing the registrar getting ready to give me Valium just in case I panicked. His hand was shaking as he filled the syringe. The whole thing was horrible. I remember being wheeled down to theatre. It seemed like I was watching a scene from a medical program.

Now I was in theatre and they were anaesthetising me, pricking my legs to see if they would twinge or not, indicating that the epidural was working. They then pinned this screen that had pictures of little duckies all over it in front of me so I couldn't see what was happening. Richard was scrubbed up and had to sign a piece of paper saying he wouldn't stand up.

They did manage to turn the baby with the forceps and thankfully let me try to deliver her by myself. It was easy. Although I couldn't feel a thing, I finally managed to push our baby out in three pushes (after that long, difficult, 38-hour labour!).

Richard stood up and was shouted at to sit down, but he had managed to see the baby.

'Ah, it's a little girl,' he said.

When I heard Richard's words, I threw off my oxygen mask and tried to sit up. I then saw this little slithery thing covered in blood, lying on my stomach crying, and I was so happy.

'Is she all right?' I asked twice. I was so frightened something might be wrong with her.

'She is fine,' came the reply.

They took my baby to the other side of the room for about three minutes, cleaned her up and wrapped her in silver paper. They then put this little parcel onto my chest. I just looked at her. I didn't know what to do. Richard said, 'Kiss her.' I did kiss her, but it felt funny. Then they took her away again.

I found out later that she had been taken outside to Mum, who was waiting outside the theatre while I was stitched up. I was cut and had torn, and they had cracked my coccyx with the forceps.

Eventually I was in my ward and Richard brought me our baby, where I put her straight to my breast. She was gorgeous and I was so excited. Geraldine weighed 3865 grams and was 51 centimetres long.

My midwife had stayed with me throughout my entire ordeal, right up to that time where I thought I was going to die. I was made to feel like the most important person in the world by my mum, my midwife and Richard.

For some reason, I couldn't believe I could produce a perfect baby, but Geraldine is more than perfect – she is divine. She makes my life easier, not harder.

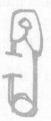

Breech birth

A baby may present in a breech position – that is, where the baby's bottom or more rarely a foot or knee is at the opening of the uterus (cervix) rather than the baby's head. When a woman is 28 weeks pregnant, there is a 25 per cent chance that the baby will be in a breech position. As the pregnancy progresses, the baby usually turns so that its head tips down. When a woman is full term, around 3 to 4 per cent of babies remain in the breech position. Some methods used to encourage breech babies to turn head-down include massage, homoeopathy, exercises using gravity and external cephalic version (ECV), where a doctor tries to turn the baby through the mother's abdominal wall. However, some babies are destined to stay in the breech position. If this is the case, a decision is made as to how the baby will be born. If there are no problems, a breech baby can be born vaginally. The labour will be monitored carefully, with a midwife or doctor skilled at breech birth providing assistance.

Jeannie's second birth story

Jeannie

Waking at about 5 am to go to the toilet, I noticed a big, bloody show. Concerned at how bright the blood was, I hoped and assumed my labour would start soon, but as yet there was still no pain.

Three weeks earlier and 35 weeks pregnant, the doctor had told me at my antenatal checkup that this baby was a footling breech, but would probably turn by the time I was in labour. Now, three weeks later (two weeks before the baby's due date), the blood was upsetting me. A feeling of panic swept over me. I hadn't had a show with my first baby, so didn't know if this blood was normal. I went in to wake up Joe, who was sound asleep and snoring. 'I think I'll be going into labour soon,' I told him, then explained what had happened with the blood.

Joe was now wide awake and I was still feeling panicky, so we decided to phone the hospital. 'There is no need to rush, but come in when you can,' we were told. So, bundling up Melissa, our four-and-a-half-year-old daughter, Joe and I took her to Mum's place, then headed to the hospital.

The midwives and doctor took a urine sample, examined me, then took an X-ray of my pelvis. Next they told me the news: our baby was still a footling breech and I also had placenta praevia. I would probably need a caesarean.

I hoped the doctor would tell me there was a chance they could turn the baby, but he said that because of the position of the placenta it wasn't possible. My placenta was lying right across the birth entrance. The doctor was also convinced that the bleeding was not due to a show but from the placenta beginning to break away from my uterine wall. I was told to go straight to another hospital, a 30-minute drive away, as our local hospital didn't have a maternity wing.

We arrived at about 9.45 am. I was admitted straightaway and checked by ultrasound, after which a monitor was strapped across my stomach to measure the strength of my contractions. But I had had no contractions, which is what I kept telling the midwives. Regardless of this, the monitor was kept on and, for the next three hours, I listened to the baby's heartbeat.

Soon I was given some lunch. Great, I thought, feeling much relieved; if they are going to give me lunch, they probably won't be giving me a general anaesthetic, or a caesarean.

About an hour after lunch, the doctors came to tell me about the trial of labour they had planned. They were going to see if I could have the baby without a caesarean. The thought of a trial of labour absolutely terrified me, as I knew the baby was still a footling breech, so I lay worrying about it for nearly an hour, picturing myself giving birth to a baby doing the splits bottom-first.

Next the doctors came back and told me they weren't going to do the trial of labour after all, but would be performing a caesarean section. Just those words 'caesarean section' terrified me.

At 4.30 pm, the midwives put me onto a trolley and made me feel comfortable. They wheeled me to the procedure room. Two drips were inserted into my hand, after which I lay there for about twenty minutes. I was so scared I was shaking, and could actually see my heart pumping.

A doctor came back all dressed in green and tried to reassure me. Then I was wheeled into theatre, where I lay for a few minutes watching them hook me up and run around. I don't think I missed a thing! I looked at all those machines and was never so scared in my life. I even thought I was going to die. 'Where is my husband?' I asked. (Everything was so foreign that I needed someone familiar to be with me.) Joe finally did come in, but I didn't recognise him because he was dressed in green, the same as the doctors, and had white cloth boots on. The doctors then positioned Joe on one side of my head and told him not to move. I looked at Joe for reassurance, as I needed to know everything was going to be all right. But he was just as worried as I was!

Machinery was all around me – heart monitors, plastic bags to pump air and, in the corner of the room, that piece of equipment used to start your heart! This was the final straw for me. I'm a goner and I'm going to die, was all I could think. Then a nurse whisked a black mask over my face as the anaesthetist slowly pushed anaesthetic in through the drip in my hand. 'You'll be asleep in a couple of seconds,' he said. I also heard the nurses say, 'We'll see you soon.' Then I just caught the anaesthetist's last words: 'When you wake up, you'll have a new...'

Christopher was born at 5.46 pm. As I was waking up, I could feel them stapling me. It was burning and I couldn't move! I couldn't even move my eyelids!* I must have gone back under, because the next thing I knew I was waking up in recovery. My main aim was to get the mask off, as I felt it was suffocating me. But I was so weak it took me ages to lift my hand to flick it off. Then, just as I managed to get the mask off, the nurse came in and put it straight back on!

One hour later I was wheeled back to my bed. Everything was fine and Joe was waiting for me. Once in bed, I was told I had a little boy who weighed 3215 grams and was 51 centimetres long.

The doctor came in just before our baby was brought in. 'You've got a very happy husband,' he said. 'When they delivered your baby and told your husband it was a boy, he made a fist, jumped off his chair into the air, and cried out, "Yes!".'

Soon they brought our baby in to me. He had lots of red hair and big brown eyes. He was just perfect! I felt wonderful. Everything I had been through was worth it, and I was just so happy to have our little boy.

Jane's first birth story

I was 35 weeks pregnant and had found out the previous week that my baby was breech. My doctor had tried unsuccessfully to turn him twice. He then referred me to a specialist, who tried again, unsuccessfully. He did an internal examination and said it wouldn't be long until the baby arrived.

By the time I got home I was feeling some discomfort, as well as feeling sick. I lay down on the lounge to get some rest. Moments later my waters broke with a gush. I couldn't believe it was happening. I was at home with my teenaged sister, Karen, and my parents were away. A neighbour took Karen and me to the hospital.

Once I'd booked in they took me to a room to see how things were going. It was 5 pm and they hooked me up to a monitor. I was having contractions but I wasn't feeling them yet. After an internal examination

---

* Hospitals now have special equipment to let the anaesthetist know if a patient is coming to consciousness during an operation.

they declared that I was 2 centimetres dilated. Nothing much was happening; only light contractions that I could just feel. My sister went home.

At about 10 pm I was sent down to X-ray to have a pelvimetry to see if my pelvis was large enough for the baby's head to pass through. At this stage the contractions were stronger, but not regular. The X-rays showed that everything was okay, so it was decided to let me try to give birth to the baby in the breech position.

Nothing much was happening at midnight, so they decided I should try to get some sleep. They gave me some sleeping tablets. As soon as I tried to sleep, the contractions started to become quite strong and were regular.

I was moved to a delivery room at 2 am, as things were moving along quite well. I was coping with the pain. I rang my sister, who was to be my support person, to come in. At 4 am, everything stopped. I managed to grab about half an hour's sleep. I was very tired and only getting the occasional contraction. I was trying to walk around as much as I could but I was hooked up to a monitor most of the time. I was growing to hate the monitor. I'd had three showers and found they were great. They made me feel heaps better, but again they were limited because of the monitor.

At 6 am they decided to induce me to get the contractions going again – yet another intervention. My idea of natural childbirth had flown out the window. I proved much too sensitive to the drip. My contractions didn't stop: the peaks kept getting higher, and there were no breaks. I somehow managed to breathe through this, but the drip had to be stopped. I kept going by myself for an hour, but again the contractions nearly stopped.

They did another internal examination at about 10 am and I was 6 centimetres dilated. The specialist came in and told me in no uncertain terms that if I wanted a vaginal birth I had to do exactly what he said. This took me down a few pegs. Nothing was happening as I'd expected. He told me I was going to have an epidural and be induced again. When it was time to deliver the baby I was to be in stirrups, have an episiotomy, then a forceps delivery. It was turning into a nightmare.

The epidural was given and the drip to induce labour was started again. The contractions started and I couldn't feel them. My mother had arrived at about 2 pm. Karen and Mum stayed with me. I was now monitored all the time. The baby had one monitor attached to his bottom. This had to be put in three times. I was bed-bound. The epidural was topped up twice, as it wore off quickly. I couldn't feel the contractions, but I could push. The third top-up didn't have any effect at all. Hot packs and breathing were the only things that got me through the pain.

At about 5.30 pm on Wednesday, I felt an incredible urge to push. I'd been told by the specialist not to push until he gave me the go-ahead. He was called in. The pain was incredible; tears streamed down my face. I couldn't cope with the urge to push any longer. I had to push, but I was told to wait. It was agonising. The specialist arrived and did an examination. He said that I wasn't quite ready. I felt out of control and extremely tired. Nothing could alleviate the pain. The specialist came back and said it was okay to push when I wanted to. But by now it was so difficult because I was exhausted.

They put my feet in stirrups and heaps of people arrived – doctors, nurses and onlookers. I felt like a sideshow. I remember trying to push, but I couldn't feel anything happening. It was like an uphill battle. Then I felt the most painful burning sensation. His foot came first; the other foot was near his head. His body was relatively easy to deliver compared with the head. I wanted to scream. I let out a noise and the doctor told me to shut up and concentrate on delivering the baby. It seemed to take ages to deliver the head. It was like pushing against nothing. Joshua came into the world and was placed straight onto my tummy at 7.26 pm. He was so tiny and perfect. They took him away to check him. Moments later he was back with me, along with a bag to assist him with his breathing.

Lack of information or choice, premature labour, medical crises and insensitive care all conspired against the active birth and the positive start to mothering I had wanted. Even though the birth was difficult, it was the most precious moment of my life. I couldn't believe the emotions that overtook me. I was so enthralled by Joshua that I hardly noticed the fancy needlework they were doing on me. Joshua suffered a few problems, being five weeks premature, but it wasn't long before he overcame them.

Premature birth

For a variety of reasons, some women go into labour early. Sometimes the mother may have been advised that there may be a chance of early labour, while others must deal with it as an unanticipated emergency. Stress, illness or an incompetent cervix are some of the reasons for early labour. The signs and symptoms of early labour are the same as for full-term labour. They may proceed normally or may require a caesarean birth.

If you think that you are in early labour, contact the hospital as soon as possible. If the waters have not broken, it is occasionally possible to slow down or halt a premature labour if the labour has not been caused by a problem requiring the immediate birth of the baby. Bed rest is often the only answer to prevention of a premature birth. Women identified at risk may need to enter hospital or have complete rest at home for some time before their baby is born.

Medical science continues to make breakthroughs in the ability to keep premature babies alive and born free of longstanding problems. Babies born as young as 24 weeks have survived to come home to their parents. The most common problem occurring with such babies relates to underdeveloped lungs. Depending on the baby's condition at birth, premature babies often require a ventilator (a tube inserted into the lungs attached to a machine to breathe for the baby). The babies are sent to neonatal wards where they live in humidicribs and have highly specialised attention. Some remain there for only a few hours or days, others stay for weeks or even months. It is a difficult and challenging time for parents.

One of the hardest things for parents of premature babies is not being able to hold or feed their child. Staff encourage parents to be with the baby as much as is practicable, and there is much rejoicing when the baby goes home.

If you go into premature labour and your hospital does not have specialised neonatal facilities, you will either be transferred to a hospital with such facilities or a team will come to take the baby to such a hospital after the baby is born.

Shantiel's birth story

I was having a normal pregnancy with morning sickness, and then at 27 weeks my waters broke. I rang the ambulance and was rushed to hospital, where it was confirmed that my waters were ruptured. I was in a small country hospital so I was told they would have to transfer me to a larger hospital with a neonatal unit. I was terrified, as I didn't think my baby would survive. I didn't know anything about premature babies and I was a blubbering mess. I was given an injection of betamethoizone, which is a drug to help develop the baby's lungs. They inserted a drip and organised an ambulance to transfer me to the Mater Mother's Hospital in South Brisbane.

By the time I arrived at the hospital I was having contractions and was very scared. The doctors told me the baby's chances of surviving were 40 to 50 per cent. They gave me an injection to try to stop the labour. I rested a while and prayed a lot, and the contractions eventually stopped. They told me the longer they left my baby in utero, the better its chance of surviving. I was taken to the prenatal ward and had to have total bed rest. I continued to leak fluid over the next four days and had contractions on and off.

On my fourth day in hospital, things went from bad to worse. Early in the evening they came to check the baby's heartbeat and movements. The nurse looked really worried after examining the monitor report. She said she needed to see the doctor straight away. She was gone for five minutes but it seemed like an hour, as I knew something was terribly wrong. The doctor came in and listened to my baby's heartbeat. He then said he needed to take some blood, as he suspected that I had an infection which had spread to baby. This meant my baby was at high risk of developing problems.

Then my nightmare became reality. The doctor came in telling me the baby had to come out immediately. Suddenly the room was filled with nurses prepping me for a caesarean. I was unprepared for a C-section, as I had had three normal births prior to this. An anaesthetist came to tell me they needed to give me a general anaesthetic, as it was an emergency, and that it would happen in ten minutes. The nurses put in more drips and prepared me for surgery. I was rushed to an operating theatre and it was off to sleep for me.

I woke up in recovery and the nurses told me I had a little boy weighing 1171 grams. He was only 28 centimetres long. They wheeled my bed into the nursery to see him – this tiny, tiny little baby boy. We named him Nicholas. Then they took me to my room. I woke the next morning not really remembering having seen my baby. The nurse was great. She told me a little about him and showed me two photos. They then got me in a wheelchair and took me up to see my little boy.

The doctors told me he was on a ventilator and that he was a very sick boy and probably wouldn't make it. He had respiratory distress and pulmonary emphazima (PIE). I was scared for him and me. He was so perfect; everything was there except that his lungs hadn't developed yet. He was so sweet and innocent lying there fighting to live.

As the days went by, he got worse. He was given a brain scan and I was told he had had an intraventrical haemorrhage.

A few days later he started to improve. After seven weeks in the intensive care unit he came off his ventilator. They transferred him to the special care nursery – this was a huge step. It had been a long haul. I didn't get to hold Nicholas until two weeks after he was born. Then it was only for five minutes, as he was so sick. After that I only got to hold him once a week. I expressed my milk for him. It was so hard. It was like he was not all mine and I had to ask to do anything for him.

When Nicholas was eight weeks old we were transferred to Toowoomba Hospital, which was a little closer to home. After four weeks, all Nicholas needed apart from oxygen was to learn to feed from me and get fat. We were getting organised to go home, as babies on oxygen can still go home. The doctors decided to try him off the oxygen one last time. They had tried about twenty times before, but this time, to our delight, he was okay without it. We roomed in with him on the ward for two more days, and exactly twelve weeks and two days after his dramatic entry into the world, we took him home.

Nicholas has developed well. He is a lovely seven-year-old boy now. The doctor had told me they didn't expect him to survive. He was so sick and tiny, and now he is so healthy and full of life.

After Nicholas I had five other premature babies, all at different weeks' gestation. Dylan was 28 weeks and 1234 grams and was given only a 1 to 2 per cent chance of survival. He developed PIE and his left lung shut down, but he made an incredible recovery. The doctors were amazed. He came home after nine weeks in hospital. Alexander was fifteen weeks early. He only weighed 851 grams when he was born. He developed PIE and died when he was four days old. Then we had Jack, who was thirteen weeks early and weighed 1171 grams. He was very sick and it was touch and go for seven weeks. He came home after ten weeks. Samantha was seven weeks early and weighed 1351 grams. She was always a well baby and only needed to get fatter and learn to feed. She spent five weeks in hospital. Then last of all I had Sophie. She was five weeks early and 1710 grams. She had a little breathing trouble at first and was taken by helicopter to Royal Brisbane Hospital. She was in hospital for only four weeks.

All my prems were born by caesarean section. A premmie baby is hard on the mother, father and the family. It is the biggest roller-coaster of all. For many weeks you don't know from one day to the next whether your baby will be there the next day. It has been hard, but I love all my children. My only advice to someone who has a premature baby is to be with it as often as possible. It's your baby and he or she knows you are there. Babies do so well when they know you love them. It's a long haul, but in the end it's all worth it. You will take home your beautiful baby.

Best wishes.

Multiple births

Labouring with multiple babies is essentially the same as for single births, although there may be more intervention after the first baby. However, you and your babies will be monitored closely, with constant checks on the fetal heartbeats and the positions. As mentioned before, multiple births are usually premature. Often this is only by a few weeks, with labour often commencing for twins around 36 weeks of pregnancy. If the woman does not go into labour by 37½ weeks, some obstetricians prefer to induce the birth as they consider it safer.

The greatest concern is for the second twin, for whom birth may be delayed and who may show signs of distress. The second twin's head may be high up and the obstetrician may have to manipulate the baby into the birth position. To ensure contractions are maintained, Syntocinon may be used, even if the birth has not been induced. Most obstetricians will insist on a hospital birth where they have access to operating theatres in case of the need for a caesarean section. However, normal births are possible and occur in at least half of all twin births.

Jen's twins

Jen had been delighted to find she was having twins. Her story continues from Part 1.

By 37 weeks I was finding it difficult to lie down for too long because of the pressure on my heart, and was becoming a little fed up with the tiredness and the waiting. At 37.5 weeks I was preparing to go out for dinner at around 8 pm when I felt this unusual pop in my stomach, followed by a major gush – one of my waters had broken (the twins were fraternal so therefore had separate placentas and sacs). Contractions then started immediately and were very close together. Andy and I went straight to the hospital and were admitted into the labour ward so they could monitor the babies' heartbeats. The monitoring became a bit of a concern, as one of the heartbeats kept on disappearing because Twin B (as he was known at that stage) was not keeping still. After much fiddling, the obstetrician decided he would concentrate on getting the babies out rather than worrying about finding heartbeats, so by 9.30 pm I had had an epidural, was on a drip having Syntocinon and was sitting back enjoying the attention. Everything then went like clockwork until my final epidural top-up just as Twin A's head was crowning at around 12.30 am. Up until then I had been able to push and feel the sensation of bearing down, but I no longer had any feeling and the contractions stopped. Twin A's head was sucked back in. They then had to externally manouevre Twin A's head down and use a ventouse to suction him out. Twin A arrived at 2 am.

They then broke my second waters and repeated the procedure for Twin B, who was born twenty minutes later.

I had two beautiful healthy boys, each weighing exactly 2880 grams. The whole experience was amazing. I was thrilled that everything went so smoothly and that I didn't have to have a caesarean. Then the afterpains began. No one had warned me how excruciating they were. Because of the twin pregnancy, I was given Syntocinon after the delivery to speed up the contracting of my uterus in order to reduce blood loss. This contracting caused the afterpains, which I found to be similar to my labour pains. These lasted on and off for around 24 hours, but were severe only for the first hour while I was still getting Syntocinon, and while I was breastfeeding. Everything else happened as it had with the birth of my first son. I felt fantastic at being able to bend over, lie down comfortably and, most of all, finally wrap my arms around my four beautiful boys.

Jasmine's birth story

Jasmine was surprised to discover she was having twins. Her story continues from Part 1.

Thirty-seven and a half weeks came, and I just couldn't wait for it to be over. I hoped my labour would start naturally, without the need for an induction. Although I had heard a lot about inductions, I didn't really know what to expect and was very worried about it.

B-day arrived. Mum came down to our home to look after Charlie and Nicole. As George and I waved goodbye, six-year-old Charlie was crying and waving back. I felt a sense of impending change and sadness leaving behind our two children, but I was also looking forward to the pregnancy being over.

We arrived at the hospital at 8 am. My doctor arrived at 8.30 am and gave me an examination. I was discovered to be 8 centimetres dilated already, even though I was not yet in labour. The doctor explained that he was going to prepare me for an epidural block but would not yet start the drugs to numb me. The drugs, he said, could be quickly administered in case of the need for an emergency caesarean. He then explained that the obstetrician needed this to be done before the induction started, as it was a lot easier to do if I was not already experiencing contractions.

The epidural took fifteen minutes to insert. I had to be curled on my side with the two midwives and George holding me down so that I wouldn't move. It was very painful.

My obstetrician arrived and the induction was set up. My waters were broken at the same time. Within seven minutes of these procedures I was in full-on labour, with no mild, crampy contractions to begin with. These severe pains were coming every three minutes, with each contraction lasting one and a half minutes. After a short time, the obstetrician had to leave the room and said, 'Beep me if anything happens, I'm just going into the wards to check on someone.' He had only been gone for about ten minutes when I suddenly felt the desperate urge to push. The midwife and doctor checked me, to discover the first baby's head! So the obstetrician was called back in.

'I've got to push. I've got to push,' I kept saying. My doctor replied by pointing his little finger at me, saying, 'Now don't you push – not yet.' The obstetrician came back and I had to be flat on my back while I was strapped down and my feet put in stirrups. 'No, no,' I said. Both doctors looked panicky and said, 'Don't push until we are ready for you.' Once strapped down I was asked to push.

'You're doing very well,' my doctor said with a great big smile. 'You're doing great,' he kept repeating reassuringly. But the obstetrician had an almost permanent worried look on his face, as if he was expecting something to go wrong. And I had to cooperate with him implicitly.

It was now 10.40 am. With the next contraction, I pushed and our first baby started to come out. I was then asked to stop pushing while the baby's mouth was cleared. This was also to minimise tearing. Once again I was told to push, during which time the whole head came out. Then, with the next contraction, I gave one hard push and out came the baby's shoulders, followed immediately by the rest of the body. All I could see was my doctor's smiling face saying, 'You've done it. You've got one out!'

They cut our little girl's cord. She was crying. They then put her into a little see-through cot next to my bed. All I could see were these two beady little eyes staring at me. It was wonderful.

We then had to get the other baby out, which turned out to be a little more difficult. Baby number two's head was still up high. There were a few panicky minutes while my stomach was manipulated to bring our baby down. After this was done, I had to push as hard as I could with the next contraction. The baby's head came half out, then once again I had to stop pushing while the baby's mouth and throat were cleared. With the following contraction, the obstetrician said, 'Now get this baby out all at once. No waiting for the next contraction, just keep pushing until the baby is out.'

Four and a half minutes later, out came our second baby. By this time I was feeling really ill. The doctors put our babies onto my stomach for a few minutes, but I felt as though I had just delivered a bus. Both babies tried to suck, but the first-born had trouble grabbing the nipple. Baby number two had no trouble at all.

'You are very fortunate,' my doctor said to me. 'You have two healthy babies who are both very strong.'

I had known from my three ultrasounds that I was having twin girls, but George had had less faith in the ultrasounds. He was surprised when he had learned they were both girls.

'Well, you've got your two girls,' my husband said.

I still had to give birth to the placenta. It was enormous, and felt like having another baby. I felt great relief when it was finally over. I had no stitches and no tearing. Over the next hour, I felt quite ill. I was cold and shaking all over. More blankets and electric blankets were added to my bed. I knew I was losing a lot of blood. The girls were taken away to be weighed and measured.

Simone (the first-born) weighed 2494 grams and was 50 centimetres long; Danielle was 2947 grams and 52 centimetres.

Finally the girls were brought back all wrapped in little hats and gloves (to prevent further temperature loss). They looked so cute and funny. Now our family was complete, with one boy and three girls. We couldn't have been happier!

Kuini's third story – the home birth of her twins

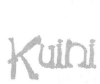

Kuini had an extremely difficult and emotional time during her pregnancy. She had also become convinced that her second twin would be stillborn. Her story continues from Part 1.

The day I started to go into labour I was one week overdue and as usual had a yearning to be near trees and grass. I went for a walk and sat on the grass just listening to and enjoying the rustling of the trees. It was now that I thought, 'Yes, I'm ready to give birth.'

I was lying on the floor and rolled over and my waters broke. It was about 10 pm. I began house cleaning, with Pat helping me clean the bathroom and make up the bed ready for the birth. Then around midnight we phoned the midwife, who came over two hours later. She gave me an internal examination and discovered I was dilating well. In fact, I was 9 centimetres already, and as with my previous labours I hadn't experienced any painful contractions.

Not long after this, the midwife gave me a second examination. She wanted to force the final centimetre of dilation. It was extremely painful and I said, 'But I'll be finished dilating in ten minutes or so – what's the problem with that?' I then became very annoyed and asked her to please leave the room. (Of course the midwife and I have since discussed this, as she was very hurt at the time. But I just wanted a peaceful birth, and because this was my third labour, I wasn't too shy to ask for what I wanted.)

When the first baby's head started to crown, the midwife came back into the room. When Hamish was born at 3.20 am, out popped this huge pink baby, weighing 3741 grams. The midwife had previously thought I would have a small baby because of the trauma I had been through.

It was a really lovely birth, but I was now absolutely exhausted. I had my beautiful baby in my arms and I just couldn't be bothered giving birth to another baby. So I simply crossed my legs. I just wanted to rest for ten minutes. But the midwife, through her medical knowledge, was urging me to have the other baby.

'Please give me ten minutes to catch my breath,' I said. So I took my time to gather my energy. The whole affair of shifting country, moving repeatedly, a relationship break-up and so on must have really taken their toll. I was extremely exhausted – spiritually, physically and emotionally.

One hour later I was finally ready to give birth, but my contractions had stopped. I was just like a dead battery. So there we were, Pat, the midwife and myself, just sitting on the bed trying to figure out how to get my contractions going again. Then I thought, 'Well maybe we'll put the first baby, Hamish, onto my breast.' This was successful. My baby would suck and a contraction would happen. He would be removed and I would then bear down. My baby would suck, and another contraction would happen. And so it went on until Jamie was born.

As soon as he came out, I knew he was dead. He was very white, and very, very cold. The midwife placed him on my stomach. He was so rubbery, it was as though he didn't have any bones. Jamie and I lay down and the midwife used her fingers on his chest to give him CPR. She breathed life into him about three times while I massaged his legs. It was then that he opened his eyes. Absolutely thrilled, I now put my baby to my breast where he sucked immediately. So we now had two beautiful boys. It was just fantastic!

As it turned out, my twins were born weighing 3741 grams and 2834 grams. Then there were their two separate placentas. No wonder I had looked so big and everyone had been staring at me!

The midwife was absolutely shocked by Jamie's condition at birth – even three years later when we talked about it. Jamie is a very cheeky little boy, extroverted and so full of life. He loves to sing and dance but is also very delicate and shy under all that bravado. I just love him so much, as I do all my children, and feel very fortunate to have him.

Older mothers

A woman is considered to be an 'elderly primagravida' in obstetric terminology, or an older first-time pregnant woman, if she is more than 35 years of age. The average age of mothers in Australia has now crept up to 29.1 years, and a small percentage of the total are in their forties. Almost 45 per cent of all new mothers are more than 30 years of age.

While figures show that there is a greater likelihood of intervention in the labours of older mothers, if a woman of 35 years or more is in good health, having taken care of herself while pregnant and received proper nutrition, there is no reason why she can't have a problem-free, normal birth.

Sharlit's first birth story

I was 40 years old and had been married to Melesm only two months when I suspected I was pregnant. I went for a check-up and was overjoyed when the doctor congratulated me on being pregnant. 'It's almost a miracle,' was how the doctor put it, to which I replied, 'This baby was an answer to prayer.'

For the first three months I was sometimes a little depressed. I would cry for no reason and became nervous quickly. I also vomited some mornings and didn't have much of an appetite, but I forced myself to eat for the sake of our baby. After three months I developed an appetite and ate just about everything! I was happy through the rest of the pregnancy.

At four months, I had friends who were at the same stage of pregnancy as myself and their babies were quite active, whereas mine didn't move much. This concerned me greatly, so I often prayed to God to make my baby normal.

I developed diabetes at seven months, which was carefully monitored. At the check-up the doctor told me my baby's head had already engaged, and said, 'You never know, maybe you could deliver soon.'

Around this time I also began having pains between my legs. In the eighth month the baby's head went up again and the problem lessened. When I entered the ninth month I was sent for a check-up to see if the baby's head had engaged again. The new doctor wasn't sure, but said she thought it had. By now it was becoming even more difficult to sleep than it had been. In the last days, even sitting became painful because of the baby's head under my ribs. (I could feel it with my hands!)

On the day of the birth my membranes ruptured at 10 am. I had no pain or contractions, so I rang the hospital and went in. By 6 pm I still had no contractions. I had a shower and it happened at last: I had my first contraction. This was soon followed by contractions coming at a steady pace at intervals of half an hour, then fifteen minutes, then ten minutes, then five. At 8 pm they took me to the delivery suite where they discovered the baby had not turned and its head was not down — its bottom was! They asked if I wanted an injection for pain relief and were talking to each other about whether or not I would need a caesarean. I asked my husband about the injection, saying, 'What do you think?' Then we both said together, 'Let's pray'. Soon Meslem suggested that I not have the injection, as he thought it might make our baby sleepy and prolong the labour. Someone then told me it was too late to have the injection – I was fully dilated. God had answered our prayer.

Before long I had the urge to deliver our baby. I was now in second stage and the nurse was asking me to bear down – but nothing was happening. Soon the doctor said, 'The baby's heartbeat sounds slow. Please help us to save the baby and try your best to push while I put my fingers around the baby's hips to pull him out.'

I wasn't sure what was happening, but suddenly it felt as though my insides were coming out as the doctor tugged on the baby. The baby received a slight injury on his bottom and was still not completely out. So I was given two small cuts and our baby was delivered.

Our son was born and he was beautiful! His leg was dislocated from the hip and his heartbeat was erratic, so he was whisked away to the special care nursery where he remained for five days. I went to see him every opportunity I had, and breastfed him when I could. We were allowed to take him home when he was five days old and I continued to breastfeed him until he was six months old.

Joshua Gandjou was born weighing 3300 grams, healthy, happy and beautiful, after a four-hour labour (which they said wasn't bad for a first baby). We couldn't measure his length, however, because of the dislocated hip. The doctor advised us to sleep Joshua on his back. By the time he was four months old his hip had healed without treatment.

Joshua is now nine months old and beginning to crawl, and I am pregnant with our second child. It is wonderful being a mum!

Carol's ninth birth story

One week before my due date I was preparing to post a parcel and buy a few things at the corner store. I had six of our eight children with me. A strong, continuous lower back pain came over me. By the time we returned home an hour later, I felt very weak and started shaking. I also felt nauseous and I could no longer prepare lunch, or even bend over to pick things up. I contacted the hospital and the midwife informed me, after learning that I was 37 years old and having my ninth baby, to come in for a check-up.

Clem took me to the hospital. I still wasn't experiencing any contractions, but I was told I was probably in early labour. My cervix was very soft and 2 centimetres dilated. I was also told they were going to admit me, as my blood pressure was 150/90 with protein present in my urine. A fetal heart monitor and uterine trace showed regular painless contractions, so something was happening.

I phoned my friend Debbie to ask her to pray for me. 'I'll pray they don't intervene and that you are interfered with as little as possible,' Debbie promised.

I went to the toilet and discovered lots of bright-red blood. The nurse wasn't in the least concerned. 'It's just a show and means you'll probably start labour sometime this week,' she said.

But I wasn't reassured, as although I had had shows with most of my other labours, none had been this bloody. Nevertheless I determined in my heart to trust God, regardless of my feelings.

Overnight my blood pressure rose to 150/100, so it took the hospital staff some convincing to allow me to return home.

The next day the contractions continued all day until they were coming every ten minutes apart, although they were still not painful. But by 5 pm I suspected true labour might start very soon. Since most of my labours had been fast (one or two hours from first pain to delivery), I suggested to Clem he take me to the hospital to avoid painful labouring during a mad rush. Clem phoned his twenty-year-old niece, Mandy, and as soon as she arrived to look after the children, Clem and I left for the hospital. Just before we left I phoned my friend Debbie and asked her to pray that the baby not be born until June (which was only four hours away), as our family already had a birthday in every month except January, June and July! But these contractions didn't progress to true labour anyway, although once again I was admitted into hospital with high blood pressure and protein present in my urine. Happily, a trace showed the baby happy, well and kicking heaps. But once again I had to talk hospital staff into letting me go home the next day (as my blood pressure rose still further during the night). While waiting for the staff to let me go home, I had a fruitful discussion with a young woman who was 34 weeks pregnant with her first child and having a lot of problems. The baby's heartbeat was too slow and the baby wasn't growing as it should have been.

On examination the next day by my doctor, I was found to be still 2 centimetres dilated and my cervix soft. My blood pressure was still raised, and after I commented that Clem was sick of it all, the doctor said, 'I'm working at the hospital tonight all night until morning. Come in any time and I'll break your waters to start the labour.'

We were ready to leave for the hospital after a lovely family meal made by Clem's brother, Robin, who had come to babysit.

So Clem left me in the capable hands of the hospital staff, expecting to come back later to some baby action. In the meantime, I read God's word and started praying. A strong feeling came over me that what I was doing might not be God's will. I prayed, 'Please Lord, don't let them break my waters if this is not your will. Let your will be done for the birth of this baby. I think I have done the wrong thing in coming here; please can you turn the situation around for good.'

A short while later, at my doctor's request, the head midwife was called to examine me. 'We are not allowed to let you go home,' she informed me. 'With blood pressure of 90–100/130–160, you'll be staying here until you have the baby.'

I was still only 2 centimetres dilated when I was taken to the first-stage labour ward to wait to have my waters broken. I informed Clem of the risks of interfering in God's timing for the birth. I felt that the breaking of my waters could cause the prolapse of the cord, meaning an emergency caesarean to save the baby. Consequently, when the doctor finally arrived to break my waters, Clem wouldn't let him do it. But the doctor wouldn't let me go home because of my blood pressure. So it was back to the same hospital bed and the 34-week pregnant woman. She was keen to share prayers with me.

Early Saturday morning my doctor came to see me, looking very tired and apologising that my waters hadn't been broken. 'Don't worry about it,' I told him. 'I've had friends praying that I have no unnecessary intervention, so you can't fight God.' I then added, 'If it's okay I'd like to go home, and I'll try not to come back again unless I'm actually in heavy labour.' So my doctor agreed and I went home a couple of hours later.

It was now Saturday and I had gone to bed at about 7 pm. Just before I'd fallen asleep I had cried and prayed to God, telling Him I was sick of everything and please could He start my labour as soon as possible. Five hours later I was awoken by a contraction. After 25 minutes I knew this was the real thing. Clem panicked when he saw that I was truly in labour, and wouldn't wait for his friend Tony, who was to babysit, to arrive. Instead he woke up our eldest daughter, Amanda (thirteen), and had her babysit our sleeping children until Tony arrived. Happily, we passed Tony on his way to our place, so I could relax about the children. But Clem didn't relax. 'Do you mind if I go through red lights?' he asked me.

'Yes I do mind,' I replied, telling him the sad story of the couple who had been killed in a car crash on their way to the hospital to have their fourth baby, leaving their children as orphans.

Arriving at the hospital for the fourth time in six days, Clem and I rather sheepishly approached reception, putting up with, 'Are you here to stay this time?' But I'm sure the receptionist knew I was, as she witnessed one of my contractions. An examination showed me 3 centimetres dilated. Hurray — something was finally happening! It was approximately 1 am, and by 2.30 am I was already 8 centimetres dilated. I had remained upright, hugging onto Clem during most of my contractions.

Every eight minutes or so I had to lie down to have a fetal heart monitor placed against my stomach. It certainly made contractions during this time very painful. In fact, it got so bad that every time the midwife got out the monitor I screamed a little in protest and anger, anticipating the more severe contractions about to come. Also during these extra painful contractions I could hear another woman screaming from the pain of her labour, so I prayed for God to take away our pain quickly.

Shortly after that, Clem and the midwife lifted me upright on the bed, into a pile of pillows and a beanbag (at my request), and my pain halved. I now began pushing with every contraction. Five minutes later, at 2.49 am, the baby was born. The midwife asked me if I wanted to see my baby, so I turned around and saw I had delivered a girl. I was ecstatic. Lily Jean Barbar, our seventh daughter, weighed 2940 grams, was 50.5 centimetres long and had a head circumference of 33.8 centimetres.

The next eleven minutes saw me deliver the placenta without Syntocinon. And then there was more time spent holding, admiring and breastfeeding my baby while Clem made numerous phone calls to his parents, brothers and sisters and their families. Also to Tony back home looking after our children.

Eventually I had a shower and was sent down to the ward holding Lily in my arms as the midwife pushed me in a wheelchair. Nothing can describe the pure joy of this experience.

The woman I had prayed for as I was having my own very painful contractions was in the same hospital room. I discovered two people had also lifted her upright (although she hadn't even asked for it), and twenty minutes later she had given birth quickly and without tearing, just as I had.

Much joy has been experienced in our family because of Lily's arrival. Our children all adore her, including two-year-old Christine, who said to me the day before I gave birth, 'Mummy, can I have a baby girl?'

Debbie sent me this Bible verse when she found out I had delivered a little girl and had named her Lily. 'I am the rose of Sharon and the lily of the valleys. As a lily among thorns is my love among the daughters.' (Song of Solomon 2:1–2)

Breastfeeding

Being able to breastfeed your baby is such a wonderful experience. It is a special time for mother and baby where the closeness helps them to bond. Yet breastfeeding is something that new mothers and their babies need to learn how to do together.

There is always an abundance of advice on hand for new mothers attempting to breastfeed, especially from women who have done so themselves successfully, but this can often be overwhelming if you are having problems.

Hospital midwives, having seen many women breastfeed, are often keen to offer their support, too. Unfortunately, in some hospitals with a large staff and many staff changeovers, advice can be conflicting. To try to overcome this, most hospitals are attempting to ensure that one method is taught and passed on to breastfeeding mothers.

Colostrum

Colostrum is a yellowish liquid produced by the breast. It contains many nutrients and is your baby's ideal first food. It also contains properties to help raise your baby's immunity levels and help resist infections.

Women have colostrum in their breasts from the sixteenth week of their pregnancy. Some women actually leak colostrum later in their pregnancy. Colostrum is ready for your baby from the moment he or she is born. (This includes women who have caesarean births.) The earlier you breastfeed your baby following the birth, the earlier your milk is likely to come in. Colostrum turns into transitional milk after about three days, then into mature milk, and although the timing differs from woman to woman, this process usually takes about three weeks.

Frequently, mothers experience hungry babies who are not content with the amount of colostrum supplied. This can contribute to teary-eyed mothers anxious about their baby's health before their larger quantity of mature milk comes in. Alternatively, some babies are very sleepy during this two- to three-day period and are quite content with the amount of colostrum they receive. Just because you do not have large amounts of colostrum does not mean you will not have plenty of breast milk by day three. One way to ensure your full supply comes in is to nurse your baby whenever she or he wants to – even if you believe they are not getting much. Babies (both breast- and bottlefed) often lose up to 10 per cent of their birth weight during this period but normally regain the weight before they are two weeks old.

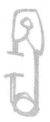

Very full breasts and engorgement

At around two to five days after birth, the breasts start to fill with milk. This is known as the milk coming in. The breasts usually become very full and tight, and often feel enormous and uncomfortable. Very full breasts are caused by a combination of the breasts rapidly filling with milk, and an increase in blood supply, which is necessary for milk production. Very full breasts usually last for a couple of days. Frequent breastfeeds are the best way to relieve it. The baby should be placed on the opposite side from which the last feed occurred, as this ensures equal stimulation and emptying of the breasts. If it is difficult for the baby to attach to the breast due to fullness under the nipple, a little milk can be expressed using either your hand or a breast pump. Expressing a small amount of milk will soften the nipple and make attachment to the breast much easier. Discomfort can be managed by placing cabbage leaves (preferably refrigerated ones) on the breasts. The cabbage leaves should be changed when they become limp or every two hours, and should be removed once the breasts are comfortable.

Engorgement is painful condition where the breasts become hard, red and shiny. It occurs when the breast tissue becomes swollen and blocks the milk ducts, decreasing the milk flow from the breast. Fortunately, engorgement is not a common condition. Strategies to relieve engorgement are the same as those used to relieve very full breasts. Other strategies include placing warm compresses on the breast just prior to breastfeeding, as well as gently massaging the breast in a circular motion, paying particular attention to any lumpy areas. Assistance from a midwife or lactation consultant may be required.

Breastfeeding positions and avoiding nipple pain

It is important that you feel comfortable with breastfeeding. If you are anxious, self-conscious or experiencing other strong emotions about it, this may upset your baby and affect your milk supply, exacerbating your difficulties.

It is essential that your baby be correctly positioned while you breastfeed, since an improperly attached baby can create problems. For example, your child may be prevented from receiving enough milk, or you may experience painful, cracked nipples. The following is one correct way to practise holding your infant to ensure correct positioning at the breast.

1 Take hold of your baby.

2 Turn the baby onto its side, putting its head level with your breast.

3 Now hold the baby so you are looking down at its shoulders and hips. Its whole body and face should be turned towards you.

When holding your baby like this, there is a technique you can use to open your baby's mouth, and that is to stroke the baby's nose and lips with your nipple. The infant should open its mouth, and when it does, pull your baby in against your breast with your arm. Your baby should now be in a correct position to nurse.

Fair-skinned people have to be even more careful with correct positioning, as their skin is a lot more sensitive and they are more prone to nipple pain.

Another way to prevent sore nipples is to change nursing positions frequently.

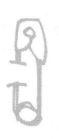

Nipple soreness

Nipple soreness is a common problem experienced by most women in the early days of breastfeeding. Strategies to reduce the incidence of nipple soreness include:

- Making sure that the baby is correctly latched onto the breast. The baby should be held closely and should have a large amount of the areola (this is the dark area surrounding the nipple) in its mouth. The baby cups the breast with its tongue.
- Expressing a small amount of hind milk at the end of each feed, patting it onto the nipple and areola, and then allowing the nipple to air dry.
- Avoiding plastic-backed nursing pads.
- Wearing a well-fitting bra.
- Exposing nipples to the air or briefly to sunlight.
- Ensuring that the suction the baby has on the breast is broken before removing the baby from the breast (this can be done by inserting a clean finger into the corner of the baby's mouth).
- Seeking the advice of a midwife or lactation consultant if there are any problems. Most difficulties are resolved with support, correct advice and perseverance.

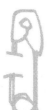

Tips

You should be as comfortable as you can while breastfeeding to help you relax and encourage milk let-down. This may not be easy in the first days following delivery due to stitches, afterpains, a caesarean delivery or just plain nerves at being new to it all, but all things should improve as you recover from the birth.

If you wish to increase your milk supply, try breastfeeding more frequently – every two to three hours. If your baby is not keen to breastfeed this often, express milk instead. Also ensure that you are getting enough rest and that you are eating a well-balanced diet.

If you are having trouble with a plentiful supply and a small baby who needs a slower flow, try lying down to breastfeed, as this can limit the speed at which your milk flows. Pillows placed under your arms and/or baby, to lift him or her higher, can help make breastfeeding this way more comfortable.

Glossary

Amniotic fluid

The liquid that surrounds and protects the baby and is contained within the amniotic sac.

Amniotic sac

A thin, transparent membrane that holds the baby in the amniotic fluid, the amniotic sac is commonly known as the bag of waters.

Anaesthesia

Partial or complete loss of sensation that occurs when an anaesthetic is administered.

Apgar score

Whether your baby is born in the hospital or at home, he or she will be given Apgar scores to determine his or her condition. A newborn baby can score a maximum of 10 points. The scores are usually done twice, at one and five minutes following birth. If the baby's condition is poor, the Apgar score may be repeated at ten minutes after birth. (See table on page 188.)

Artificial rupture of the membranes (ARM)

The amniotic sac (or membranes) are broken with an instrument and amniotic fluid is released. This is usually done to induce labour or to speed labour up.

Birth stool

A specially designed stool that the mother can sit on during labour and while giving birth. It permits the woman to give birth in an upright position.

The Apgar score

	Points
HEART RATE	
Absent	0
Less than 100 beats per minute	1
More than 100 beats per minute	2
RESPIRATION	
Absent	0
Slow, irregular	1
Regular, crying	2
COLOUR	
Blue, pale	0
Body pink, extremities blue	1
Completely pink	2
MUSCLE TONE	
Limp, flaccid	0
Some flexion of limbs	1
Active	2
REFLEX RESPONSE	
None	0
Minimal, grimace	1
Crying, cough, sneeze	2

Braxton Hicks contractions

Usually painless, irregular contractions of the uterus that occur from the third month of pregnancy. May be confused with the contractions of true labour.

Breech presentation

This is where the baby's buttocks and legs present at the pelvis rather than the head. The woman can experience difficulty giving birth if the baby is in a breech presentation, particularly since the baby's head does not have time to mould. If attempting a vaginal breech birth, it essential to have present a doctor or midwife experienced in breech births. An episiotomy (birth cut) is often performed during a breech birth in order to widen the vaginal entrance.

Caesarean section

A major surgical operation to remove a baby from its mother's uterus. A caesarean section is done by making an incision through the woman's abdominal wall and uterus.

Caput

This is a small swelling on part of the baby's head as a result of pressing on the cervix during labour. It is harmless and will disappear within a few days.

Carpal tunnel syndrome

This is pins and needles and numbness in the fingers and hands. It is caused by fluid retention (oedema) which presses on nerves to the hands. It usually disappears after the birth of the baby.

Cervical suture

If the cervix is damaged or weak, a stitch or stitches are put into the cervix to keep it tightly closed to help prevent the woman going into premature labour. (*See also* incompetent cervix.)

Cervix

The cervix is the neck of the uterus. Located at the base of the uterus, it hangs down into the vagina and is the area that dilates to allow the baby to be born.

Conception

The joining of female ovum with male sperm, resulting in fertilisation.

Contractions (of the uterus)

During a contraction, the uterine muscle shortens and tightens, mostly at the top, causing the bottom of the uterus (the cervix) to open. Contractions also gradually move the baby down.

Crowning

Crowning occurs the moment the widest part of the baby's head stretches the vulval outlet. During crowning, the baby's head no longer recedes back into the birth canal when there are no contractions.

Dilation

Dilation refers to the opening of the cervix during labour. When the cervix is closed it is said to be 0 centimetres dilated. When the cervix is fully open and the second stage of labour begins, the cervix is said to be 10 centimetres dilated.

Drip (intravenous drip)

A cannula (a special type of needle) is inserted into a vein and intravenous fluids are connected to the cannula by tubing. The fluids slowly drip from a chamber (or bag) at the beginning of the tubing. This is a method by which Syntocinon is given to a woman during pregnancy to induce or speed up her contractions. The speed of the drip can be turned up or down as required. Other liquids and drugs can be administered via the drip, for example, glucose, saline solution and blood.

Eclampsia

Eclampsia is an extremely rare but life-threatening condition. If the symptoms of pre-eclampsia are not controlled, the situation becomes critical, resulting in kidney failure, convulsive fitting and possibly coma. Once the mother has been stabilised with oxygen and medications, the baby must be delivered urgently, usually by a caesarean section. In most instances, the condition resolves itself once the baby has been born.

Electronic fetal monitoring

This refers to a method of monitoring the baby's heartbeat and the woman's contractions (if she is in labour). Electronic fetal monitoring may be done externally, using two small pieces of equipment which are strapped to the woman's abdomen by large elastic belts (one monitors the baby's heart rate and the other monitors the woman's contractions), or internally (see internal fetal monitoring).

Enema

The introduction of a solution into the rectum which causes the bowel to empty. The routine administration of an enema to a woman in labour has no benefit.

Engorgement

Two to five days after birth, the breasts fill rapidly with milk, which causes them to increase greatly in size. If the breasts are not adequately emptied, breast tissue presses on milk ducts and can actually block these ducts. Engorgement is a very painful condition in which the breasts become hard, red and shiny. This condition is greatly relieved when the baby feeds or milk is expressed by hand or pump. A hot shower or icepack can also greatly relieve the pain of engorgement.

Epidural anaesthesia

A procedure where anaesthetic is introduced into the epidural space (located over the spinal column), causing numbness or loss of sensation from the waist down.

Episiotomy

An episiotomy, also known as a birth cut, is a cut made to create a wider outlet to aid the delivery of the baby. The incision is made into the woman's perineum (the area between the vagina and anus) after she has been given a local anaesthetic.

If the woman's perineum is unable to stretch sufficiently during the crowning of the baby's head, it may tear. This is not necessarily a bad thing, as a tear will often heal better and with less pain. Yet many doctors believe that an episiotomy is easier to repair than a tear, which is why some doctors routinely perform one.

If the woman is exhausted after a long labour and unable to push her baby out, an episiotomy might be needed to help the baby emerge. An episiotomy is often carried out when the doctor needs to use forceps to deliver the baby.

Helping and holding the woman into a standing position can provide the same assistance as an episiotomy and is a much better option, if possible.

Face presentation

Where the baby's head is extended backwards and the baby's face presents at the opening of the cervix.

First stage of labour

First stage of labour is said to begin when there are regular contractions and the cervix begins to open. First stage ends when the cervix is fully open or has reached 10 centimetres dilation.

Forceps birth

Forceps consist of two separate spoon-shaped blades, which are placed on either side of the baby's head and locked together to assist with the birth. They permit force to be applied by a doctor, while protecting the baby's head at the same time.

Fundal height

The distance between the top of the pubis symphysis (public bone) and the top of the uterus. The fundal height is measured and recorded during pregnancy to follow the growth of the baby.

Gestational diabetes

Approximately 3 per cent of pregnant women develop gestational diabetes. Most women do not notice any symptoms, so health-care practitioners encourage pregnant women to have a glucose tolerance test when they are about 28 weeks into their pregnancy to determine whether they have this condition. Gestational diabetes is managed primarily by following a healthy diet with the assistance of a dietitian. Some women, however, may need to take insulin. Once the baby is born the condition usually disappears.

Incompetent cervix

A rather unfortunate name to describe a cervix that is weak or has been damaged and therefore not able to remain firmly closed during pregnancy. This can increase the risk of miscarriage or premature birth because the cervix cannot hold the fetus in the uterus as it grows bigger. One or two stitches can be inserted into the cervix to help overcome these problems. These are removed before labour.

Induction

An induction is a series of one or more procedures that artificially start labour.

One method of induction is using a prostaglandin gel or pessaries, which are inserted into the vagina. This is usually done during the evening, causing contractions to begin overnight or by morning. The prostaglandin acts by duplicating the natural events that lead to labour.

Another method of induction is artificial rupture of the membranes (ARM). This is done with an instrument resembling a crochet hook, which is inserted into the uterus to make a small hole in the membrane so the waters can escape.

A third method of induction is the use of the drug Syntocinon (often used in combination with ARM). This is a synthetic form of the natural hormone oxytocin, which your body produces in the posterior pituitary gland. When Syntocinon is administered during labour, it requires you to be attached to a drip. This particular method of induction often produces a faster, more intense labour. Syntocinon is often injected into your thigh as your baby's shoulders are being born to help your uterus contract and bring on a speedy delivery of the placenta.

Internal fetal monitoring

During labour, a small fetal electrode may be attached to the infant's head so its heartbeat can be heard. This is done by penetrating a small section of the head, enabling a monitor to be attached. This procedure can only be done when the mother's cervix is 2 to 3 centimetres dilated and her membranes have ruptured.

Internal monitoring is extremely accurate, which is why it is used. It is able to detect the baby's heart rate and pick up problems the infant may be experiencing. Doctors can then decide whether or not to intervene with an emergency caesarean. There is a risk of infection with this monitor, and some babies will be born with a temporary bruise or rash where the electrode was placed.

Meconium

This tar-like, dark substance is a baby's first bowel motion. Sometimes a baby will pass meconium in the amniotic fluid before birth. This can indicate that the baby is or has been in distress.

Midwife

A person who is educated in the art and science of caring for women through pregnancy, birth and beyond.

Moulding

The bones of a baby's skull do not fuse together until after the birth. This allows the head to be moulded slightly as it comes through the birth canal to make birth easier. At birth, a baby's head may look elongated or slightly pointed, but this will change after the birth and the head will become rounded in appearance.

Natural birth

A natural birth is a normal vaginal delivery without the use of instruments (such as forceps) or drugs for pain relief. Because all drugs the mother takes during her labour will enter the baby's bloodstream via the umbilical cord, many women prefer to use natural methods to control their pain, such as hot water and breathing exercises.

Nitrous oxide

A gas that is mixed with oxygen and is inhaled using a mouthpiece or mask. Commonly known as laughing gas, nitrous oxide can be used for pain relief during labour.

Obstetrician

A surgeon who specialises in complications during pregnancy, birth and beyond.

Oxytocin

Oxytocin is a natural hormone which the body produces in the pituitary gland (located in the brain). It causes the uterus to contract during labour. Synthetic oxytocin (Syntocinon) is used to induce labour or speed up delivery.

Perineum

The skin and muscle located between the vagina and the anus.

Pethidine

A synthetic narcotic drug, in the same family as heroin and morphine. Pethidine can be used for pain relief during labour.

Placenta

The placenta is commonly known as the afterbirth. It is the placenta which enables the baby's circulation and its mother's circulation to pass closely together, allowing an exchange of nutrients from mother to baby, and also returning the baby's waste back to its mother. The mother's and baby's blood do not mix. During pregnancy, the placenta is attached to the wall of the uterus and is delivered after the baby is born.

At term, a healthy placenta looks like a piece of raw liver. It is about the size of a dinner plate and is normally brownish-red in colouring.

Placenta praevia

The placenta is normally attached to the upper section of the uterine wall, but, in the case of placenta praevia, it is implanted in the lower section instead. The placenta now lies in front of the baby's entrance to the birth canal. An indication that this is happening is if the mother passes blood, usually in the last trimester of her pregnancy. In severe cases where the placenta is completely blocking the cervix, a caesarean section is needed for the baby's safe delivery. In less severe cases, where only a small part of the placenta is touching the cervix, a vaginal delivery may be possible.

Pre-eclampsia (toxaemia)

This is a condition occurring during pregnancy where the mother experiences raised blood pressure, protein in her urine and usually swelling of her extremities. Bed rest, treatment with drugs or an early birth may be necessary.

PUPPP

Pruritic urticarial papules and plaques of pregnancy is an itchy rash which forms on stretch marks on the stomach in later pregnancy and can spread over the body. It is extremely uncomfortable but is not harmful to the mother or baby. It disappears slowly after the birth.

Rupture of membranes

This is the tearing or breaking of the membranes (sac) that contains the amniotic fluid, resulting in the leaking of amniotic fluid. The most common time the membranes rupture naturally is at the end of the first stage of labour or into the second stage of labour. In approximately 10–15 per cent of cases the membranes will rupture before labour begins.

Sacrum

The sacrum is a wedge-shaped bone that is part of the spinal column. The sacrum is situated on the bottom of the lumbar vertebra and above the coccyx, forming the back wall of the pelvis.

Second stage of labour

The second stage of labour begins when the cervix is fully dilated and ends with the birth of the baby. It is during this stage of labour that a woman pushes with the contractions.

Show

This is the bloodstained mucous plug that comes away from the cervix when it is beginning to stretch at the start of labour.

Strep B

A bacterial infection known as Group B Streptococcus (GBS), which 10 to 30 per cent of women carry in their vaginal or rectal areas. GBS commonly returns after treatment with antibiotics. Women who carry GBS and have another risk factor are more likely to have a baby with a GBS infection after birth (a very serious condition).

Antibiotics may be given to women with GBS during labour or alternatively they may only be given if the mother has GBS and an additional risk factor (policies vary).

Syntocinon

A synthetic form of the natural hormone oxytocin. It is a medication used to induce or speed up labour and is also used to manage the third stage of labour.

Transition

The transition between the later stages of the first stage of labour and the beginning of the second stage of labour.

Third stage of labour

The third stage of labour begins with the birth of the baby and ends with the birth of the placenta and membranes.

Trial of labour

This is where labour and a vaginal birth are attempted, even though a medical condition exists which may mean that the woman has an increased risk of a caesarean section. For example, a trial of labour may be carried out in cases of pelvic disproportion (the baby's head appears to be too large to pass through the pelvis) or placenta praevia.

If no problems occur with the trial of labour, the woman will continue her labour and give birth vaginally. If problems arise, a caesarean section is performed.

Ultrasound

Ultrasound is sound produced at a very high pitch. For an ultrasound test during pregnancy, a transducer is used to pass sound waves into the body. When the sound waves encounter a structure within the body, part of the sound wave is bounced back. This echo is registered electronically and transmits onto a screen as a dot. The density of the body tissue dictates the colour of the dot. The more dense the structure, the lighter the colour of the dot. An image is formed in varying shades of white, grey and black. Ultrasound technology is used to monitor babies during pregnancy.

Uterus

The uterus is a muscular, pear-shaped, hollow organ of the female reproductive system. It is designed to hold and nourish a baby until it is fully formed and ready to be born.

Vacuum extraction (or ventouse)

Used as an alternative to forceps in assisting with the birth of a baby. A metal or plastic cup is applied to the baby's head and a vacuum is created to apply suction. Traction is applied by a doctor during contractions to facilitate the birth of the baby's head.

Vernix

A white cream that covers the baby while it is in the uterus. Vernix is produced by special glands in the baby's skin and helps prevent the baby's skin from becoming waterlogged. Some babies are born with vernix still on their skin.

Contacts and resources

The addresses below are supplied for information only and are not recommendations by the publisher or the author. It is the responsibility of the reader to access services on contact with organisations and individuals.

Breastfeeding

Australian Lactation Consultants
Lactation consultants offer support and assistance to women with breastfeeding difficulties. Names of lactation consultants in different areas are available from the Lactation Resource Centre
Phone (03) 9885 0855

Australian Breastfeeding Association
National Headquarters
1818–1822 Malvern Road
East Malvern VIC 3145
PO Box 4000
Glen Iris VIC 3146
Phone (03) 9885 0855
Fax (03) 9885 0866
Email: nursingm @nmaa.asn.au
Web: www.breastfeeding.asn.au

For any breastfeeding mothers experiencing difficulties, please contact the Breastfeeding Association's 24-hour telephone counselling service:
ACT & Southern NSW (02) 6258 8928
New South Wales (02) 9639 8686
Northern Territory (08) 8411 0301
Queensland (07) 3844 8977 or (07) 3844 8166
South Australia (08) 8411 0050
Tasmania (03) 6223 2609
Victoria (03) 9885 0653
Western Australia (08) 9340 1200

Karitane (NSW only) (*see* Parenting support)

Lactation Resource Centre
Established by Australian Breastfeeding
  Association
Provides up-to-date information on
  breastfeeding.
PO Box 4000
Glen Iris VIC 3146
Phone (03) 9885 0855
Fax (03) 9885 0866

Tresillian Family Care (NSW only) (*see* Parenting Support)

Caesarean support

Birthrites
Provides information on caesareans and vaginal birth after caesarean, with Australia-wide contacts.
C/A 4 Leavis Place
Spearwood WA 6163
Phone (08) 9418 8949
Web: www.birthrites.org

The Maternity Coalition Inc.
Email: inquiries@maternitycoalition.org.au
Web: www.maternitycoalition.org.au

Childbirth education

Childbirth Education Association (Brisbane)
PO Box 206
Petrie QLD 4502
Phone (07) 3285 8233
Fax (07) 3285 8233

Childbirth Education Association (Darwin)
PO Box 42162
Casuarina NT 0811
Phone (08) 8927 2575

Childbirth Education Association (Alice Springs) Inc.
PO Box 542
Alice Springs NT 0871
Phone (08) 8952 5353 or (08) 8953 3876

Childbirth Education Association (NSW) Ltd
PO Box 413
Hurstville NSW 2220
Phone (02) 9580 0399
Fax (02) 9580 0399

Childbirth Information Centre (Tasmania)
Information on options for birthing
156 Warwick Street
Hobart TAS 7000
Phone (03) 6231 0633

Resources and Information Centre (Hospital and Home Birth)
Minnawarra House
Armadale SA
Phone (08) 9479 1413

Cot death

(*see* SANDS and SIDS* under Grief and loss)

Gastric reflux

Vomiting Infants Support Association (VISA) of NSW Inc.
PO Box 4105
East Gosford NSW 4105
Phone (02) 4324 7062
Fax (02) 4324 7062

Reflex Infants Support Association (RISA) of QLD Inc.
PO Box 1598
Fortitude Valley QLD 4006
Phone (07) 3229 1090

Grief and loss

SANDS* (Stillbirth & Newborn Death Support Group)

ACT
Building 5, Canberra Hospital
PO Box 11
Woden ACT 2606
Phone (02) 6244 2372

NSW (*see* SIDS* NSW)
Phone (02) 9721 0124
Fax (02) 9681 5954
Email: sandsnsw@ozemail.com.au
Website: www.sandsnsw.org.au

QLD
PO Box 1730
Office/drop-in centre
45 Candell Street
Auchenflower QLD 4066
Phone (07) 3217 7882 (24 hours/seven days)
Fax (07) 3217 8334
Email: sandsqld@ezyweb-tech.com.au
Website: www.powerup.com.au/~sandsqld/

SA
PO Box 380
Parkholme SA 5043
Phone (08) 8277 0304

TAS
PO Box 786
Rosny Park TAS 7018
Phone (03) 9517 4470

VIC
Suite 208/901
Whitehorse Road
Box Hill VIC 3128
Phone (03) 9899 0218
Email: info@sandsvic.org.au
Website: www.sandsvic.org.au

WA (*see* SIDS* WA)

* SIDS (Sudden Infant Death Syndrome) and SANDS have merged in NSW and WA into one organisation called SIDS. Calls to SANDS in WA and NSW will be diverted to SIDS in those States for two years from the date of this book's publication.

SIDS* (Sudden Infant Death Association
  Australia)

National SIDS Council of Australia Ltd
  (Administration only)
Level 1, 891 Burke Road
Camberwell VIC 3124
Phone (03) 9813 3200
Fax (03) 9813 3099
Email: national@sidsaustralia.org.au
Website: www.sidsaustralia.org au

ACT
PO Box 3118
Weston ACT 2611
Phone (02) 6287 4255
Fax (02) 6287 4210
Email: canberra@sids.australia.org.au

Hunter region
SIDS Hunter region
PO Box 64
The Junction NSW 2291
Phone (02) 4969 3171
Fax (02) 4969 3170
Email: newcastle@sidsaustralia.org.au

NSW
PO Box 379
Guildford NSW 2161
Phone (02) 9681 4500 or 1800 651186
Fax (02) 9681 5954
Email: sydney@sidsaustralia.org.au

NT
GPO Box 3414
Darwin NT 0801
Phone (08) 8948 5311
Fax (08) 8948 5244
Email: darwin@sidsaustralia.org.au

QLD
PO Box 241
Mt Gravatt QLD 4122
Phone (07) 3849 7122 or 1800 628 648
Fax (07) 3849 7121
Email: brisbane@sidsaustralia.org au

SA
301 Payneham Road
Royston Park SA 5070
Phone (08) 8363 1963 or 1800 656 566
fax (08) 8363 2829
Email: adelaide@sidsaustralia.org.au

TAS
2 Spring Street
Burnie TAS 7320
Phone (03) 6431 9488 or 1800 625 675
Fax (03) 6431 6081
Email: tasmania@sidsaustralia.org.au

VIC
1227 Malvern Road
Malvern VIC 3144
Phone (03) 9822 9611 or 1800 240 400
Fax (03) 9822 2995
Email: melbourne@sidsaustralia.org.au

WA*
33 Sixth Avenue
Kensington WA 6151
Phone (08) 9474 3544 or 1800 199 466
Fax (08) 9474 3636
Email: perth@sidsaustralia.org.au

Home birth (*see also* Midwifery services and Childbirth education)

Birthplace Support Group Inc. (and Fremantle
  Community Midwives)
80 Canning Highway
Fremantle WA 6158
Phone (08) 9319 8043
Email: midwives@iinet.net.au

Darwin Home Birth Group Inc.
PO Box 41252
Casuarina NT 0811
Phone (08) 8948 2373
Fax (08) 8981 5841
Lisa Moore (08) 8948 4731
Marion Lejeune (08) 8948 2121

* See footnote on p. 199

Home Birth Access Sydney
PO Box 66
Broadway NSW 2007
Contact Robyn Dempsey
Phone (02) 9888 7829
Website: www.homebirthaccess.sydney.com.au

Home Birth Australia
PO Box 1085
Byron Bay NSW 2481
Contact Sue Cookson
Phone 1800 222 180 or (02) 6680 2717
Website: www.homebirthaustralia.org

Home Birth Network of SA (Inc.)
PO Box 7
Collinswood SA 5081
Contact Sally Amazon
Phone (08) 8388 5659

Home Midwifery Association (QLD)
PO Box 655
Spring Hill QLD 4000
Phone (07) 3839 5883

Midwifery services (*see also* Home birth *and* Childbirth education)

Australian College of Midwives

ACT
GPO Box 1918
Canberra City ACT 2601
Phone (02) 6286 8094
President: Emma Baldock
Phone (02) 6249 6764

NSW
PO Box 62
Glebe NSW 2037
Phone (02) 9281 9522
Fax (02) 9281 0335

NT
PO Box 4178 1
Casuarina NT 0811

QLD
PO Box 8073
Woolloongabba QLD 4102
Phone (07) 3366 7641

SA
PO Box 1063
Kent Town SA 5071
Phone (08) 8364 5729

TAS
GPO Box 2022
Hobart TAS 7001

VIC
11127 Grattan Street
Carlton VIC 3053
Phone (03) 9349 1110
Email: acmivic@webrider.net.au

WA
PO Box 553
Subiaco WA 6008

Australian Society of Independent Midwives

NSW
PO Box 4013
Denistone East NSW 2112
Phone (02) 9888 7829

NT
Marj Foley
Mobile Midwives
PO Box 246
Parap NT 0804
Phone (08) 8932 4759
Email: mjfoley@bigpond.com

SA
Marijke Eastaugh
29 Robinson Road
Meadows SA 5201
Phone (08) 8388 3146 or (08) 8393 1758
Email: marijke@charior.net.au

TAS
Annie Popelier
(available for home birth)
Phone (03) 6239 6699 or (03) 6223 5348

Pregnancy, Birth and Beyond
27 Hart Street
Dundas NSW 2117
Phone (02) 9873 1750
Email: janepalm@rivernet.com.au
Website: www.pregnancy.com.au

Independent Midwife Terry Stockton
27 Wentworth Street
South Hobart TAS 7004
Phone (03) 6231 0633 (day)
Phone (03) 6223 5348 (night)

Melbourne Midwifery
Robyn Thompson
PO Box 247
Altona VIC 3018
Phone (03) 9398 2020
Mobile 0418 324 058
Website: www.melbmidwifery.com.au

Midwifery and Natural Childbirth Centre
Susan Jane
336 Oxford Street
Leederville WA 6007
Phone (08) 9242 3330
Mobile 0417 942 301

Western Australian Community Midwifery Program
A government-funded program to supply midwifery care and home birth care for 150 births per year.
PO Box 1336
Fremantle WA 6959
Phone (08) 9339 0021
Email: communitymidwifery@iinet.net.au

Parenting support
Baby Health Centres
These centres are listed under 'Early Childhood Health Centre' in your local telephone book.

Contact Incorporated (Project for Isolated Children)
Information and referrals for parents and carers of children 0–5 years.
1st floor
30 Wilson Street
Newtown NSW 2042
Phone (02) 9565 1333

Karitane
Care for mothers and babies. Provides support, guidance and information to families, professionals and the community.
24-hour care line:
Sydney metropolitan area (02) 9794 1852
Outside Sydney 1800 677 961

Mitchell Street (corner The Horsley Drive)
Carramar NSW 2163

Randwick Family Care Cottage
146 Avoca Street
Randwick NSW 2031

Family Care Cottage
100 Murphy Avenue
Liverpool NSW 2170

Jade House
130 Nelson Street
Fairfield Heights NSW 2165
24-hour counselling line:
Phone (02) 9794 1852 or 1800 677 961

INgida Family Resource Centre
Parenting services for years 0–6.
9 George Street
Kensington WA 6151
Phone (08) 9367 7855

Playgroup Association

NSW
4/181 McCredie Road
PO Box 567
Guildford 2161
Phone (02) 9632 8577
Fax (02) 9632 6445

NT
PO Box 41405
Casuarina NT 0811
Phone (08) 8985 4968

QLD
396 Miton Road
Auchenflower QLD 4066
Phone (07) 3371 8253
Fax (07) 3870 0569

SA
47 Manton Street
Hindmarsh SA 5007
Phone (08) 8346 2722 or 1800 681 080
Fax (08) 8340 2201

TAS
PO Box 799
Launceston TAS 7250
Phone (03) 6223 4814

WA
PO Box 61
North Perth WA 6006
Phone (08) 9228 8088
Fax (08) 9228 3203

VIC
346 Albert Street
Brunswick VIC 3056
Phone (03) 9388 1599
Fax (03) 9380 6733

Tresillian Family Care Centres
(Royal Society for the Welfare of Mothers and
  Babies)
Provides positive, practical advice and guidance
on caring for babies.
Head Office
McKenzie Street
Belmore NSW 2192
Phone (02) 9787 0800
Fax (02) 9787 0880
Email: trisillian@tres.cant.cs.nsw.gov.au
24-hour parents helpline:
Sydney (02) 9787 5255
Outside Sydney and ACT 1800 637 537

Wanslea Family Services
Family care and support.
110 Scarborough Beach Road
Scarborough WA 6922

Postnatal depression
Karitane (*see* Parenting support)

Helen Mayo House SA
226 Fullerton Road
Eastwood SA 5063
Phone (08) 8303 1183

**PaNDA (Post and Antenatal Depression
  Association Inc.)**
PaNDA offers support, reassurance and information
to women experiencing postnatal depression.
90 High Street
Northcote VIC 3070
Admin and support line (03) 9482 9400
Fax (03) 9482 9420
Email: panda@vicnet.au
Web: www.vicnet.au/~panda/

Canterbury Family Centre
1st floor
19 Canterbury Road
Camberwell VIC 3124
Phone (03) 9882 5396
Support contact (03) 9882 5756
Fax (03) 9813 2203

PND Personal Support Network ACT
PO Box 366
Curtin ACT 2605
Phone (02) 6286 4082 or (02) 6288 8337

PND Therapeutic Parenting Group
TAS
232 Newborn Road
Newtown TAS 7008
Phone (03) 623 3 2700

Post Natal Depression Group WA
c/- G. Spiers
2 Albatross Court
Heathridge WA 6027
Phone (08) 9401 2699

Postnatal Depression Therapy Group
NSW
St John of God Day Services
13 Grantharn Street
Burwood NSW 2134
Phone (02) 9747 5611

Preconception care

Foresight Association
The Association for the Promotion of
  Preconceptual Care
The Secretary
124 Louisa Road
Birchgrove NSW 2041

Pregnancy and birth organisations

AIMS (Australia) Inc.
The Association for Improvement in Maternity
Services (Australia) deals with any complaints
women may have with their maternity care. It
supports the rights of parents to choose the place
and manner of birth, the rights of parents to
accurate information, and the parents' right to
be treated with respect during pregnancy and
childbirth.
PO Box 420
Red Hill QLD 4059
Phone (07) 3376 4355

Australian Action on Pre-Eclampsia (AAPEC)
A voluntary organisation set up to provide
information and support for women and families
affected by pre-eclampsia.
PO Box 29
Carlton South VIC 3053
Phone (03) 9330 0441

Childbirth Information Service
156 Warwick Street
West Hobart TAS 7000
Phone (03) 6231 0633

Maternity Alliance
Maternity Alliance seeks to ensure that women
have an effective voice in all matters related to
maternity care.

PO Box 789
Artarmon NSW 2064
Phone (02) 4961 1626

Maternity Coalition Inc.
PO Box 73
Brunswick South VIC 3055
Phone (03) 9380 2863

Natural Birth Association
156 Warwick Street
West Hobart TAS 7000
Phone (03) 6231 0633

Pregnancy, Birth and Beyond
27 Hart Street
Dundas NSW 2117
Phone (02) 9873 1750
Email: janepalm@rivernet.com.au
Website: www.pregnancy.com.au

SIDS (*see* Grief and loss)

Twins or more

Australian Multiple Birth Association Inc.

ACT
PO Box 1162
Woden ACT 2606
Email: carmba@yahoo.com au
Website: www.mytech.com.au/carmba/index.html

NSW
PO Box 105
Coogee NSW 2034
Website: www.amba.org.au

NT
PO Box 42069
Casuarina NT 0811
Phone (08) 8922 8888

QLD
Phone (07) 5535 6360
Email: johnlon@bigpond com.au

SA
46 Lockwood Road
Erindale SA 5066
Phone (08) 8364 0433
Fax (08) 8364 043

TAS
PO Box 139
Prospect TAS 2750
Phone (03) 6344 6466

VIC
PO Box 914
Glen Waverley VIC 3150
Phone (03) 9857 4454

WA
PO Box 410
West Perth WA 6872
Website: http//mbawa org an

Bibliography

Banks, M. 1998, *Breech birth woman-wise*, Birthspirit Books, New Zealand.

Bennett, V. R., & Brown, L. K, 1993, *Myles Textbook for Midwives*, 12th edn, Churchill Livingstone, London.

Enkin, M., Keirse, M. J., Renfrew, M. & Neilson, J. 1995, *A Guide to Effective Care in Pregnancy and Childbirth*, 2nd edn, Oxford University Press, Oxford.

Nursing Mothers Association of Australia 1993, *An Introduction to Breastfeeding*, Victoria.

Robertson, A. 1999, *Preparing for Birth: Mothers*, ACE Graphics, Sydney.

Further reading

Pregnancy

Doctors and Staff of the Royal Hospital for Women 1999, *The Pregnancy Book*, revised edn, HarperCollins, Sydney.

Eisenberg, A., Murkoff, H. E. & Hathaway, S.E. 1990, *What to Eat When You're Expecting*, 2nd edn (Australian), Angus & Robertson, Sydney.

Eisenberg, A., Murkoff, H. E. & Hathaway, S.E. 1996, *What to Expect When You're Expecting*, 2nd edn (Australian), Angus & Robertson, Sydney.

Gillespie, C. 1998, *Your Pregnancy Month by Month*, 5th edn, HarperPerennial, New York.

Laughlin, K. 2001, *Stretching and Pregnancy*, Simon & Schuster, Sydney.

Plater, D. 1997, *How to Aim for a Successful Pregnancy after Miscarriage, Stillbirth and Neonatal Loss*, Transworld, Sydney.

Pregnancy and childbirth
Baker, R. 1997, *Baby Love*, revised edn, Pan Macmillan, Sydney.
Cook, K. 1999, *Up the Duff*, Viking, Melbourne.
Cooper, D. 1999, *Your Baby Your Way*, Random House, Sydney.
Downey, P. 1994, *So You're Going to Be a Dad*, Simon & Schuster, Sydney.
Fallows, C. 1996, *Australian Book of Pregnancy and Birth*, Doubleday, Sydney.
Kitzinger, S., 1997, *The New Pregnancy and Childbirth*, revised edn, Transworld, Sydney.
Stoppard, M.1996, *The New Pregnancy and Birth Book*, Viking, Melbourne.

After the birth
Baker, R. 1997, *Baby Love*, revised edn, Pan Macmillian, Sydney.
Fowler, C. & Gornall, P. 2001, *How to Stay Sane in Your Baby's First Year*, new edn, Simon & Schuster, Sydney.
Green, C. 2001, *Babies!*, 2nd edn, Simon & Schuster, Sydney.
Stoppard, M. 2001, *Complete Baby and Childcare*, revised edn, Dorling Kindersley, Sydney.

Websites
Birthrites
www.birthrites.org.au

Birth International
www.birthinternational.com

ePregnancy
www.epregnancy.com

Mother and Child
www.motherchild.com.au

The Maternity Coalition
www.maternitycoalition.org.au

Index